Effective Treatments for Pain in the Older Patient

Grace A. Cordts • Paul J. Christo
Editors

Effective Treatments for Pain in the Older Patient

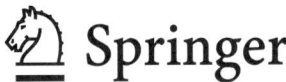

Editors
Grace A. Cordts
Optum
Complex Care Management
Pittsburgh, PA
USA

Paul J. Christo
Division of Pain Medicine
Department of Anesthesiology and Critical Care Medicine
The Johns Hopkins University School of Medicine
Baltimore, MD
USA

ISBN 978-1-4939-8825-9   ISBN 978-1-4939-8827-3   (eBook)
https://doi.org/10.1007/978-1-4939-8827-3

Library of Congress Control Number: 2018961031

© Springer Science+Business Media, LLC, part of Springer Nature 2019
This work is subject to copyright. All rights are reserved by the Publisher, whether the whole or part of the material is concerned, specifically the rights of translation, reprinting, reuse of illustrations, recitation, broadcasting, reproduction on microfilms or in any other physical way, and transmission or information storage and retrieval, electronic adaptation, computer software, or by similar or dissimilar methodology now known or hereafter developed.
The use of general descriptive names, registered names, trademarks, service marks, etc. in this publication does not imply, even in the absence of a specific statement, that such names are exempt from the relevant protective laws and regulations and therefore free for general use.
The publisher, the authors, and the editors are safe to assume that the advice and information in this book are believed to be true and accurate at the date of publication. Neither the publisher nor the authors or the editors give a warranty, express or implied, with respect to the material contained herein or for any errors or omissions that may have been made. The publisher remains neutral with regard to jurisdictional claims in published maps and institutional affiliations.

This Springer imprint is published by the registered company Springer Science+Business Media, LLC part of Springer Nature.
The registered company address is: 233 Spring Street, New York, NY 10013, U.S.A.

Preface

Pain is a very common symptom for older people. Although common, pain is often under-recognized and undertreated in the older adult. The consequences of this are a negative impact on the health and quality of life of the older adult. This book seeks to rectify this. Our hope is that this book will give the reader both a broad view of treating older people with pain and specifics on how to approach the evaluation and treatment of pain in this population.

Pain assessment and treatment is complex in the elderly. Physical, cognitive, and sensory changes can occur as we age, impacting evaluation and treatment. Multiple comorbidities and what people want for themselves as their situation changes also impact the approach to evaluation and treatment.

The book presents a variety of topics important for clinicians to understand the complexity of treating pain in the elderly. It is organized into topical chapters. Chapter 1 reviews the epidemiology of pain and the susceptibility of developing chronic pain secondary to disease and illness that older people have. Chapter 2 reviews pain assessment, discussing the complexity of the assessment needed. Chapter 3 discusses acute pain in the elderly. Chapter 4 reviews the unique physiologic changes that occur and how the changes impact evaluation and management of pain. Chapter 5 looks at specific pain conditions that affect older adults. Chapter 6 reviews classes of medications and how to use them with older adults. Chapter 7 reviews the biopsychosocial aspect of pain and reviews alternative medicine strategies. Chapter 8 discusses interventional strategies. And finally Chapter 9 discusses risks of addiction in the elderly and ways to mitigate that risk.

We believe this book will be helpful to all practitioners that care for older people: advanced practice nurses and physicians working in geriatrics and also pain specialists who may need information in treating pain in older adults.

While a book with so many contributing authors can be a long time in development, we are pleased to present it to you now. We are honored and grateful for the national authorities on pain and pain management in the elderly who have contributed to this book. We would like to thank our colleagues, students, and patients that inspired us to take on this project.

Baltimore, MD, USA Paul J. Christo
Pittsburgh, PA, USA Grace A. Cordts

Contents

Effective Approaches for Pain Relief in Older Adults 1
    Sonal S. Mehta, Erinn R. Ayers, and M. Carrington Reid

Pain Assessment in Older Adults 13
    Abisola B. Mesioye and Grace A. Cordts

Acute Pain Management in Older Adults 35
    Richard J. Lin and Eugenia L. Siegler

Unique Physiologic Considerations 53
    Nina M. Bemben and Mary Lynn McPherson

Specific Conditions Causing Persistent Pain in Older Adults 71
    Charles E. Argoff, Ravneet Bhullar, and Katherine Galluzzi

Recommendations for Classes of Medications in Older Adults 109
    Adam J. Carinci, Scott Pritzlaff, and Alex Moore

**A Biopsychosocial Perspective on the Assessment
and Treatment of Chronic Pain in Older Adults** 131
    Burel R. Goodin, Hailey W. Bulls, and Matthew Scott Herbert

Interventional Strategies for Pain in Older Adults 153
    Michael Bottros and Paul J. Christo

Assessing and Managing Addiction Risk in Older Adults with Pain 177
    Steven D. Passik, Adam Rzetelny, and Kenneth Kirsh

Index 193

Contributors

Charles E. Argoff, MD Albany Medical College, Albany, NY, USA

Erinn R. Ayers, MD Genesis Health Group, Department of Internal Medicine, Moline, IL, USA

Division of Geriatrics and Palliative Medicine, Weill Cornell Medical Center, New York, NY, USA

Nina M. Bemben, PharmD, BCPS Kaiser Permanente, Oakland, CA, USA

Ravneet Bhullar, MD Albany Medical Center, Department of Anesthesiology, Albany, NY, USA

Michael Bottros, MD Department of Anesthesiology, Division of Pain Medicine, Washington University School of Medicine, St. Louis, MO, USA

Hailey W. Bulls, PhD Moffitt Cancer Center, Department of Health Outcomes and Behavior, Tampa, FL, USA

Department of Psychology, University of Alabama at Birmingham, Birmingham, AL, USA

Adam J. Carinci, MD Division of Pain Medicine, and Pain Treatment Center, Department of Anesthesiology & Perioperative Medicine, University of Rochester Medical Center, University of Rochester School of Medicine and Dentistry, Rochester, NY, USA

Paul J. Christo, MD, MBA Division of Pain Medicine, Department of Anesthesiology and Critical Care Medicine, The Johns Hopkins University School of Medicine, Baltimore, MD, USA

Grace A. Cordts, MD, MPH, MS, CMD Optum, Complex Care Management, Pittsburgh, PA, USA

Katherine Galluzzi, DO Philadelphia College of Osteopathic Medicine, Philadelphia, PA, USA

Burel R. Goodin, PhD Department of Psychology, University of Alabama at Birmingham, Birmingham, AL, USA

Matthew Scott Herbert, PhD Clinical Psychologist, Veterans Affairs San Diego Healthcare System, Center for Excellence for Stress and Mental Health (CESAMH), San Diego, CA, USA

Department of Psychology, University of Alabama at Birmingham, Birmingham, AL, USA

Kenneth Kirsh Stoughton, MA, USA

Millennium Health of San Diego California, San Diego, CA, USA

Richard J. Lin, MD, PhD Department of Medicine, Memorial Sloan Kettering Cancer Center, New York, NY, USA

Mary Lynn McPherson, PharmD, MA, MDE, BCPS Department of Pharmacy Practice and Science, University of Maryland School of Pharmacy, Baltimore, MD, USA

Sonal S. Mehta, MD New York Presbyterian Hospital, Department of Medicine, New York, NY, USA

Division of Geriatrics and Palliative Medicine, Weill Cornell Medical Center, New York, NY, USA

Abisola B. Mesioye, MD Geriatrics and Extended Care Clinical Center, VA Maryland Health Care System, Perry Point, MD, USA

Department of Medicine, University of Maryland School of Medicine, Baltimore, MD, USA

Alex Moore Division of Pediatric Anesthesiology, Vanderbilt University Medical Center, Nashville, TN, USA

Steven D. Passik, PhD, VP Scientific Affairs, Education and Policy, Collegium Pharmaceuticals, Canton, MA, USA

Scott Pritzlaff Department of Anesthesiology, Perioperative and Pain Medicine, Stanford University, Stanford, CA, USA

M. Carrington Reid, MD, PhD Cornell Medical College, New York Presbyterian Hospital, Department of Medicine, New York, NY, USA

Division of Geriatrics and Palliative Medicine, Weill Cornell Medical Center, New York, NY, USA

Adam Rzetelny, PhD Collegium Pharmaceuticals, Stoughton, MA, USA

Eugenia L. Siegler, MD Division of Geriatrics and Palliative Medicine, Weill Cornell Medicine, New York, NY, USA

Effective Approaches for Pain Relief in Older Adults

Sonal S. Mehta, Erinn R. Ayers, and M. Carrington Reid

Growing Numbers of Older Adults and Impact on Health Care

The world's demographics are changing such that there is an ever-increasing older population. Much attention has been paid to this phenomenon in recent years, especially in developed countries [1, 2]. In 2011, the first of the baby boomers began to reach 65, and by 2030 an estimated 20% of the population will have reached this age and beyond [3]. In addition, the proportion of adults ages 80 and above will triple [4].

Pain is a highly common, costly, and frequently disabling disorder in older adults. In addition, older adults have higher rates of hospitalization, chronic diseases, and surgery which increase their risk for pain [5]. Because of these (and other) reasons, pain management in older adults has emerged as an important public health issue. This chapter reviews the epidemiology of pain and common etiologies for pain in older adults as well as its wide impact on our society. We also describe barriers to pain management and summarize both non-pharmacologic and pharmacologic approaches of its treatment in older adults.

Pain Epidemiology

Prevalence rates of pain in older adults vary from 25% to 80%. Pain is typically classified as either acute or persistent and can be due to non-cancer or cancer-related causes. Common causes of later-life pain are shown in Table 1. Acute pain is most often related to an injury or sudden onset of an illness and is highly prevalent among hospitalized older adults [6]. Persistent (also sometimes referred to as chronic) pain is defined as pain that extends beyond the expected time of healing and may or may

S. S. Mehta (✉) · E. R. Ayers · M. C. Reid
Division of Geriatrics and Palliative Medicine, Weill Cornell Medical Center, New York, NY, USA
e-mail: som9015@med.cornell.edu

© Springer Science+Business Media, LLC, part of Springer Nature 2019
G. A. Cordts, P. J. Christo (eds.), *Effective Treatments for Pain in the Older Patient*, https://doi.org/10.1007/978-1-4939-8827-3_1

Table 1 Prevalent causes of pain in later life

System	Pain source
Dermatology	Pressure ulcers, cellulitis
Cardiovascular	Advanced heart disease, congestive heart failure
Rheumatology	Gout, pseudogout, osteoarthritis, fibromyalgia, rheumatoid arthritis
Endocrine	Diabetic neuropathy
Neurology	Poststroke pain, Parkinson's disease, migraine
Infectious diseases	Herpes zoster, HIV/AIDS neuropathy
Oncology	Cancer, cancer treatments
Pulmonary	Advanced chronic obstructive lung disease/emphysema
Renal	Chronic kidney disease and end stage renal disease, nephrolithiasis
Gastrointestinal	Irritable bowel syndrome, constipation, hemorrhoids
Musculoskeletal	Low back pain, osteoporosis, costochondritis, Paget's disease

not be associated with a specific disease process [7]. Cancer pain is pain related to tissue infiltration or compression by the tumor or to the diffuse physical changes that occur related to hormones secreted by the tumor or to the diagnostic tests and treatments involved in treating the malignancy. Cancer-related pain can be either acute or persistent. For example, a breast tumor can cause acute pain locally and be treated with surgery and chemotherapy. However, chemotherapy agents may lead to persistent painful neuropathies, while surgical complications (e.g., chronic lymphedema) can also contribute to persistent pain among cancer survivors.

Approximately 50% of older adults admitted to a hospital report pain, with 20% endorsing moderate-to-severe levels of pain [6]. Cognitively impaired older adults are a particularly vulnerable population. For example, older adults with cognitive impairment admitted to the hospital with hip fractures are found to receive inadequate analgesics for moderate-to-severe acute pain [8] and less analgesics than cognitively intact older adults with similar levels of pain. Despite this knowledge and existing pain management guidelines, assessment and treatment practices vary [9], and acute pain in hospitalized older adults remains undertreated.

The prevalence of pain is also high in community-dwelling older adults. Numerous studies estimate that as many as 40% of community-dwelling older adults experience persistent non-cancer pain [7, 10, 11]. In one large cross-sectional study, the prevalence of pain in older adults was found to be 72%, and the prevalence of pain that interfered with activities of daily living increased with age [12]. Another study that sought to describe the older adult's pain experience found a prevalence rate of over 90% [13]. A particularly high prevalence of pain has been documented in the nursing home population, with up to 80% of residents experiencing persistent pain [14]. Underdetection and undertreatment of pain are most pronounced in the nursing home setting, which is especially problematic given the recent estimates that up to 42% of older persons will spend time (receiving acute and/or long-term care) in a nursing home [15]. Thus, primary care providers and specialists need to be versed in age-appropriate pain assessment and management strategies for use among older adults.

The literature on pain in later life also provides evidence for numerous patterns of pain in older adults. Studies have shown an age-related increase in the prevalence of persistent pain until the seventh decade of life, followed by a plateau or a decline in the later years [7]. In addition, when prevalence rates are stratified by pain location, the prevalence of joint pain and lower extremity pain increases with age, while the prevalence of headaches, abdominal pain, and chest pain peaks in the middle ages and then declines [5].

The aging process predisposes older adults to both acute and persistent pain (Table 1). Arthritis and arthritis-related diseases are the most common causes of persistent pain in older adults [16]. For example, osteoarthritis is one of the most common sources of pain and disability in this age group [17]. Age and obesity are major risk factors for developing osteoarthritis. Older adults are also at increased risk for acute pain problems, often occurring as a result of trauma, surgery, and non-traumatic fractures. Approximately two million joint repair/replacement surgeries (and over 700,000 vertebral compression factures) occur annually. Pain in the postoperative setting is a strong and independent risk factor for poor outcomes among older adults undergoing joint surgeries [18, 19]. Additional painful rheumatic conditions common in older adults include gout, fibromyalgia, and polymyalgia rheumatica [20].

Cancer pain is another significant source of persistent pain in older adults. Advancing age is one of the strongest risk factors for cancer occurrence [21]. Approximately 1.5 million cases of cancer are diagnosed each year in this country, the vast majority in older adults [22]. As many as 80% of persons diagnosed with cancer experience pain during the course of their illness [23], and over one quarter of cancer patients ages 65 and over with pain do not receive any analgesics [24]. Furthermore, pain that occurs as a consequence of cancer treatment (chemotherapy, surgery, radiation) is increasingly recognized as a form of persistent pain in cancer survivors [25] and complicates definitions of (and our understanding about) what constitutes cancer-related vs. non-cancer pain. Like chronic pain from other conditions, the experience of persistent pain among cancer survivors can negatively impact quality of life [26].

Age is associated with an increased burden of chronic illnesses which, in turn, increases the risk of pain. Painful neuropathies associated with diabetes and herpes zoster occur commonly in older adults and can be as, if not more, disabling than musculoskeletal pain [27]. Increasing frailty is strongly associated with pain in older adults as demonstrated by daily pain prevalence rates that range from 46% to 55% among seniors receiving home care services [28–30]. Pain is also a highly prevalent symptom occurring in the advanced stages of many chronic diseases (e.g., advanced heart, lung, renal disease and those with multiple morbidities) that are not responsive to curative treatment.

Impact of Pain in Later Life

Pain in older adults has numerous debilitating consequences affecting the individual, their caregivers, and society at large. Hospitalized older adults with a hip fracture who received less analgesics postoperatively showed higher rates of delirium, slower rehabilitation, and poor functional recovery [19]. In community-dwelling older adults, persistent pain is independently associated with physical disability, falls, depression, social isolation, poor sleep, and appetite and an overall decrease in quality of life [31, 32]. Persistent pain affects social activities and instrumental activities of daily living (ADL) and is one of the most frequently cited causes of ADL impairment among older adults [32]. In addition, persistent pain is a risk factor for poor self-rated health [33] and is associated with an increased risk of mortality [34].

Caregiving for older adults with pain is commonly provided by spouses or other family members. Chronic illnesses including pain can lead to caregiver burden and affect social and financial relationships as well as caregiver quality of life. Numerous studies have examined caregiver burden in the setting of chronic illnesses such as cancer, stroke, mental illness, and rheumatoid arthritis (RA). Recent research suggests that having an aging parent who suffers from chronic pain may have a negative impact on parent-adult child relations [35]. Furthermore, in a population of RA patients, higher rates of dependency in self-care activities were associated with higher levels of caregiver burden and increased disruption in caregiver schedules [36]. This study also found that caregivers of RA patients with pain had a higher loss of physical strength [36].

Pain costs the USA approximately $635 billion each year in medical treatments and loss of productivity [37]. One study focused on arthritis-related pain found that the health-care costs were estimated to be $81 billion annually [38]. In addition older adults with persistent pain use more health-care services than those without pain [39]. This utilization of health-care services includes multiple visits to primary care providers and specialists, a battery of diagnostic tests, emergency room visits and hospitalizations, as well as the loss of productivity of spouses or adult children caregivers.

Barriers to Pain Assessment and Management

Although pain is common and has known detrimental effects in later life, it remains underassessed and undertreated across all health-care settings. A variety of factors contribute to these age-related disparities in assessment and treatment. Impaired vision, hearing, and cognition deficits are prevalent in later life and contribute to the challenges of obtaining an accurate pain assessment. Cognitively impaired older adults in particular represent a group of older adults at increased risk for underassessment and undertreatment of pain. Manifestations of pain in this group can range from behavioral disturbances such as physical aggression and lethargy to reactions such as groaning and grimacing. These manifestations make pain management more difficult by requiring more provider time, knowledge of pain-related behaviors, and clinical judgment. A triangulated approach that includes patient self-report, observation of behaviors, and information from caregivers is recommended when assessing pain in cognitively impaired older adults [40, 41].

Older adults' beliefs about pain can serve as barriers to the assessment and management of pain. Many older adults often harbor misconceptions about pain, such as pain being a normal part of the aging process, fear of addiction, and stoic attitudes that inhibit reporting of pain and being willing to undergo treatments for pain. Furthermore, comorbid conditions and polypharmacy limit pharmacologic treatment options. For example, nonsteroidal anti-inflammatory drugs are avoided in patients with congestive heart failure and chronic kidney disease, as well as in patients on chronic anticoagulation therapy (e.g., warfarin, dabigitran). Physiologic changes related to aging affect the pharmacodynamics and pharmacokinetics of numerous drugs further complicating the management of pain in this age group. A decrease in renal function affects the elimination of drugs such as opioids and requires dose adjustment and careful monitoring for side effects.

Health-care providers contribute to underassessment and undertreatment of pain in a multitude of ways. Providers' lack of trust in patient reporting of pain and lack of routine assessments lead to inadequate pain assessments. Fear of causing harm, the subjectivity of pain, and lack of pain education on the part of health-care providers also constitute important barriers to the assessment and treatment of pain among older adults [42]. Provider lack of knowledge of pain assessment tools, medication side effect profiles, and non-pharmacologic management options further affects their ability to diagnose and treat pain effectively. Provider biases such as fear of promoting dependence and addiction, exacerbating pain-related behaviors, and legal consequences also contribute to the overall problem. Although the risk for addiction and abuse of opioids in older adults with no history of substance abuse is low, tools such as the opioid risk tool are available to incorporate routine screening for aberrant opioid-related behaviors [43]. To address the barrier of inadequate provider education, the National Institutes of Health Pain Consortium has funded 11 Centers of Excellence in Pain Education. These centers "act as hubs for the development, evaluation, and distribution of pain management curriculum resources for medical, dental, nursing and pharmacy schools to enhance and improve how health care professionals are taught about pain and its treatment" [26].

Overview of Management Approaches in Older Adults

Managing pain in older adults requires a systematic approach, starting with a thorough pain assessment, history, and exam. Multiple validated assessment tools exist to obtain information from both cognitively intact and cognitively impaired older adults. Details regarding the effects of pain on ADLs, social interactions, and mood, along with an understanding of beliefs and attitudes toward pain, are particularly important to obtain. In addition, older adults seek numerous forms of non-pharmacologic, complementary, and alternative methods of treating their pain, including nutritional supplements and chiropractors [44]. Providers should routinely ask older adults about all modalities they may have tried or are currently using and should proactively educate themselves about these treatments.

A broad spectrum of treatment options exist to ameliorate pain in older adults, ranging from non-pharmacologic methods, to pharmacologic therapies and invasive techniques. A multimodal approach can be effective and is recommended when treating pain in this age group. Non-pharmacologic methods can be classified into two major groups: physical and psychosocial interventions. Self-management programs typically combine both physical and psychosocial approaches with a goal of enhancing participants' self-efficacy to optimally manage pain and its complications. Studies focused on the effectiveness of non-pharmacologic methods in older adults are limited, and there are no clinical guidelines to recommend best practices in this population [45]. The American Geriatrics Society (AGS) recommends non-pharmacologic management as an adjunctive treatment to pharmacologic management [44]. Non-pharmacologic modalities are appropriate for a wide variety of older adults with either non-cancer or cancer-related pain, particularly those who cannot tolerate analgesics or their side effects, those at risk for polypharmacy, and those who are eager to use alternative therapies.

Physical interventions include exercise, acupuncture, transcutaneous electrical stimulation (TENS), and qigong therapy. Most of the studies evaluating these modalities in older adults targeted knee pain and low back pain [44]. Given the low cost of some of these methods, such as exercise, they should be considered early in the management of pain. Few older adults endorse using these approaches, yet they can pay substantial dividends [43, 46, 47]. Low-to-moderate exercise can increase physical function, improve joint range of motion, and slow general physical decline [48]. Movement-based therapies include aqua therapy, tai chi, and yoga. The AGS recommends that prescribed exercise programs be individualized and supervised for older adults with severe pain or physical disability. In addition, the exercise program should incorporate strength, flexibility, and endurance training.

Psychosocial interventions include self-management educational interventions, cognitive behavioral therapy (CBT), mindfulness-based meditation, and listening to music and guided imagery with progressive muscle relaxation. Self-management programs have been developed and implemented as a means of helping individuals better manage pain and other pain-related symptoms [49]. The Arthritis Foundation has disseminated the Arthritis Foundation Self-Help Program (ASHP), a community-based, pain management, and self-efficacy enhancing course [50]. Classes are taught by trained lay leaders or health professionals in diverse community settings [49]. The ASHP has been found to improve participants' pain and pain-related symptoms [51]. Several studies have found that participants sustain treatment gains over time, reinforcing the program's value [52]. Despite this evidence base, these programs have reached few US adults with arthritis or arthritis-related diseases [53]. A review of non-pharmacologic interventions found ten studies that focused on persistent non-cancer pain in community-dwelling adults aged 65 and over [44]. In summary these interventions can provide substantial benefits, including pain relief, improved coping strategies, and decreased disability during their short courses. However, research indicates that maintenance of treatment effects can be difficult. CBT, which encourages and reinforces self-management, positive health beliefs and behaviors, is recommended by the AGS for older adults with persistent pain.

A wide variety of pharmacologic therapies are available to treat older adults with pain and choosing a regimen depends on the etiology and intensity of pain, the types of co-morbidities a patient has, as well as the potential for drug-drug interactions, out of pocket costs patients have to pay, and dosing schedule. Most drug therapies can be safely initiated in older adults if these factors are taken into consideration [31]. In addition, when choosing a regimen, providers need to be familiar with the effects of age-related pharmacokinetics and pharmacodynamics.

Analgesics can be divided into three categories, non-opioids, opioids and adjuvants. Non-opioids include acetaminophen, which is often considered a first-line analgesic, and non-steroidal anti-inflammatory drugs (NSAIDS) such as ibuprofen, naprosyn and celecoxib. Acetaminophen is useful to treat musculoskeletal pain and has a mild side-effect profile. While the overall safety profile of the medication is excellent [31], acetaminophen toxicity remains the leading cause of acute liver failure in the U.S. [54]. Unintentional overdose is the leading cause of acetaminophen-induced hepatotoxicity; the vast majority of persons experiencing this outcome report having taken acetaminophen to treat their pain [53]. NSAIDs continue to be one of the most commonly prescribed and consumed analgesic agents (as over-the-counter products). Over 111 million NSAID prescriptions are written annually in the U.S. [55], and approximately 70% of older adults report taking an NSAID at least once a week [56]. While oral NSAIDs are considered more effective pain relievers than acetaminophen, this class of medications has significant limitations in the form of cardiovascular, renal, and gastrointestinal toxicity. Use of selective or non-selective NSAIDs is associated with increased risk for myocardial infarction, stroke and mortality [57].

Opioids are effective in relieving moderate-to-severe pain and can be used to treat both acute and persistent pain in older adults. Although longitudinal studies focused on the effects of opioids on older adults are limited, guidelines developed by the American Geriatrics Society support their use, along with continued reassessment of pain and medication effects. The putative benefits of treatment must always be weighed against the risks of treatment. Side effects are common (e.g., constipation, nausea, and dizziness, mental clouding) and prompt discontinuation of treatment in a substantial number of cases [58]. Furthermore, Solomon and colleagues used Medicare claims data to examine the safety of selective and nonselective NSAIDs versus opioids for non-malignant pain [59]. Subjects receiving selective NSAIDs or opioids were at increased risk for adverse cardiovascular outcomes relative to nonselective NSAID users. NSAID and coxib users had similar fracture risk, while opioid use was associated with significantly increased fracture risk, adverse events requiring hospitalization, and all-cause mortality [58]. In an effort to address the continued opioid epidemic, the Centers for Disease Control and Prevention (CDC) recently issued the *Guideline for Prescribing Opioids for Chronic Pain* to assist clinicians treating adult patients with chronic pain [60]. Finally, adjuvants include medications classified as antidepressants, anticonvulsants, muscle relaxants, and corticosteroids have been found to aid in the treatment of specific pain disorders including neuropathic pain, metastatic bone disease, and fibromyalgia.

Age is no longer a deterrent for consideration of more invasive measures to treat pain in older adults. Intra-articular injections are commonly used to treat osteoarthritis-related pain in numerous joints such as the knee and shoulder.

Hyaluronan and Hylan (also referred to as viscosupplements) are thought to work by improving the elastoviscous properties of joint synovial fluid, which progressively diminishes over time in the setting of OA. A Cochrane review [61] synthesized results from 63 trials examining outcomes in persons with knee OA. This meta-analysis found that when compared to placebo, viscosupplementation provides moderate-to-large treatment effects for pain and function, with maximal benefit detected between 5 and 13 weeks after joint injection. Epidural injections are also used as a tool in the treatment of low back pain. These procedures can be performed by a variety of providers including orthopedic surgeons, pain specialists, physical medicine, and rehabilitation physicians. Joint replacement is also available for older adults whose pain and quality of life have not improved with medications and non-pharmacologic management.

Summary

- Pain in later life constitutes a major public health problem.
- Pain is a common problem for older adults encountered across all spectrums of care from the outpatient clinics and hospitals to long-term care facilities.
- Persistent pain in older adults is associated with a decrease in quality of life as well as limitations in basic activities of daily living.
- Patient, caregiver, and provider education are key to obtaining an accurate pain assessment.
- Persistent pain in older adults requires a comprehensive but individualized approach to treatment which includes the following:
  - Assessment and reassessment of pain
  - Use of pharmacotherapy which takes into account the older adults' comorbidities and medication profile, following the adage "start low and go slow"
  - Concurrent use of non-pharmacologic modalities
  - Monitoring for side effects and impact on quality of life

References

1. United Nations. Ageing: social policy and development division. c2013. [homepage on the internet]. Available from: http://social.un.org/index/Ageing.aspx.
2. World Health Organization. WHO study on global ageing and adult health (SAGE). cWHO2013. [homepage on the internet]. Available from: http://www.who.int/healthinfo/sage/en/index.html.
3. Federal Interagency Forum on Aging-Related Statistics. Older Americans 2012: key indicators of well-being. Federal Interagency Forum on Aging-Related Statistics. Washington, DC: U.S. Government Printing Office; 2012.
4. Vincent GK, Velkoff VA. The next four decades. The older population in the United States: 2010 to 2050. US Dept of Commerce Economics and Statistics Administration. U.S. Census Bureau. 2010; p. 25–1138.
5. Gibson SJ, Lussier D. Prevalence and relevance of pain in older persons. Pain Med. 2012;13:S23–6.

6. Desbiens NA, Mueller-Rizner N, Connors AF Jr, et al. Pain in the oldest-old during hospitalization and up to one year later. J Am Geriatr Soc. 1997;45:1167–72.
7. Helme RD, Gibson SJ. The epidemiology of pain in elderly people. Clin Geriatr Med. 2001;17: 417–31.
8. Morrison RS, Al S. A comparison of pain and its treatment in advanced dementia and cognitively intact patients with hip fracture. J Pain Symptom Manag. 2000;19:240–8.
9. Mehta SS, Siegler EL, Henderson CR, Reid MC. Acute pain management in hospitalized patients with cognitive impairment: a study of provider practices and treatment outcomes. Pain Med. 2010;11:1516–24.
10. Elliott AM, Smith BH, Penny KI, Smith WC, Chambers WA. The epidemiology of chronic pain in the community. Lancet. 1999;354:1248–52.
11. Blyth FM, March LM, Brnabic AJM, et al. Estimates of the prevalence of arthritis and selected musculoskeletal disorders in the United States. Arthritis Rheum. 1998;41:778–99.
12. Thomas E, Peat G, Harris L, Wilkie R, Croft PR. The prevalence of pain and pain interference in a general population of older adults: cross-sectional findings from the North Staffordshire Osteoarthritis Project (NorStOP). Pain. 2004;110:361–8.
13. Brown ST, Kirkpatrick MK, Swanson MS, McKenzie IL. Pain experience of the elderly. Pain Manag Nurs. 2011;12:190–6.
14. Takai Y, Yamamoto-Mitani N, Okamoto Y, Hoyama K, Honda A. Literature review of pain prevalence among older residents of nursing homes. Pain Manag Nurs. 2010;11:209–23.
15. Murtagh CM, Kemper P, Spillman BC, Carlson BL. The amount, distribution and timing of lifetime nursing home use. Med Care. 1997;35:204–18.
16. Lawrence RC, et al. Estimates of the prevalence of arthritis and selected musculoskeletal disorders in the United States. Arthritis Rheum. 1998;41:778–99.
17. Anderson AS, Loeser RF. Why is osteoarthritis an age related disease? Best Pract Res Clin Rheumatol. 2010;24:15–26.
18. Williams CA, Tinetti ME, Kasl SC, Peduzzi PN. The role of pain in the recovery of instrumental and social functioning after hip fracture. J Aging Health. 2006;18:743–68.
19. Morrison RS, Magaziner J, McLaughlin MA, et al. The impact of post-operative pain on outcomes following hip fracture. Pain. 2003;103:303–11.
20. Lawrence RC, Felson DT, Helmick CG, for the National Arthritis Data Workgroup, et al. Estimates of the prevalence of arthritis and other rheumatic conditions in the United States, part II. Arthritis Rheum. 2008;58:26–35.
21. D'Agostino NS, Gray G, Scanlon C. Cancer in the older adult: understanding age related changes. Journal of GErontol Nurs. 1990;16:12–5.
22. American Cancer Society. Estimated cancer deaths by sex and age (years), 2013. [homepage on the Internet] American Cancer Society. Surveillance research. c2013. Available from: http://www.cancer.org/acs/groups/content/@epidemiologysurveilance/documents/document/acspc-037115.pdf.
23. Rao A, Cohen HJ. Symptom management in the elderly cancer patient: fatigue, pain, and depression. J Natl Cancer Inst Monogr. 2004;32:150–7.
24. Bernabei R, Gambassi G, Lapane K, et al. Management of pain in elderly patients with cancer. SAGE Study Group. Systematic assessment of geriatric drug use via epidemiology. JAMA. 1998;279:1877–82.
25. Potter J, Hami F, Bryan T, Quigley C. Symptoms in 400 patients referred to palliative care services: prevalence and patterns. Palliat Med. 2003;17(4):310–4.
26. Burton AW, Fanciullo GJ, Beasley RD, Fisch MJ. Chronic pain in the cancer survivor: a new frontier. Pain Med. 2007;8:189–98.
27. Schmader KE. Epidemiology and impact on quality of life of postherpetic neuralgia and painful diabetic neuropathy. Clin J Pain. 2002;18(6):350–4.
28. Shugarman LR, Buttar A, Fries BE, Moore T, Blaum CS. Caregiver attitudes and hospitalization risk in Michigan residents receiving home- and community-based care. J Am Geriatr Soc. 2002;50:1079–85.
29. Soldato M, Liperoti R, Landi F, et al. Non-malignant daily pain and risk of disability among older adults in home care in Europe. Pain. 2007;129:304–10.

30. Maxwell CJ, Dalby DM, Slater M, et al. The prevalence and management of current daily pain among older home care clients. Pain. 2008;138:208–16.
31. American Geriatrics Society Panel on the Pharmacological Management of Persistent Pain in Older Persons. Pharmacological management of persistent pain in older persons. J Am Geriatr Soc. 2009;57(8):1331–46.
32. Leveille SG, Fried LP. Disabling symptoms: what do older women report? J Gen Intern Med. 2002;17:766–73.
33. Mantyselka PT, Turunen JH, Ahonen RS, et al. Chronic pain and poor self-rated health. JAMA. 2003;290:2435–42.
34. Juurlink DN, Herrmann N, Szalai JP, Kopp A, Redelmeier DA. Medical Illness and the risk of suicide in the elderly. Arch Intern Med. 2004;164:1179–84.
35. Riffin C, Suitor JJ, Reid MC, Pillemer K. Chronic pain and parent-child relations in later life: does it make a difference? Family Science. 2012;3(2):75–85.
36. Jacobi CE, van den Berg B, Boshuizen HC, Rupp I, Dinant HJ, van den Bos GAM. Dimension-specific burden of caregiving among partners of rheumatoid arthritis patients. Rheumatology. 2003;42:1226–33.
37. Institute of Medicine. Relieving pain in America: a blueprint for transforming prevention, care, education and research. Washington DC: The National Academies Press; 2011.
38. Yelin E, Murphy L, Cisternas MG, Foreman AJ, Pasta DJ, Helmick CG. Medical care expenditures and earnings losses among persons with arthritis and other rheumatic conditions in 2003 and comparisons with 1997. Arthritis Rheum. 2007;56:1397–407.
39. Lavsky-Shulan M, Wallace RB, Kohout FJ. Prevalence and functional correlates of low back pain in the elderly: the Iowa 65+ rural health study. J Am Geriatr Soc. 1985;33:23–8.
40. Herr K, Coyne PJ, Key T, et al. Pain assessment in the nonverbal patient: position statement with clinical practice recommendations. Pain Manag Nurs. 2006;2:44–52.
41. Herr K, Bjoro K, Decker S. Tools for assessment of pain in nonverbal older adults with dementia: a state of the science review. J Pain Symptom Manag. 2006;31:170–92.
42. Spitz A, Moore AA, Papaleontiou M, Granieri E, Turner BJ, Reid MC. Primary care providers' perspective on prescribing opioids to older adults with chronic non-cancer pain: a qualitative study. BMC Geriatr. 2011;11:35.
43. Webster LR, Webster RM. Predicting aberrant behaviors in opioid-treated patients: preliminary validation of the opioid risk tool. Pain Med. 2005;6:432–42.
44. AGS Panel on Persistent Pain in Older Persons. The management of persistent pain in older persons. J Am Geriatr Soc. 2002;50(6 Suppl):S205–24.
45. Park J, Hughes AK. Non-pharmacologic approaches to the management of chronic pain in community dwelling older adults: a review of empirical evidence. JAGS. 2012;60:555–68.
46. Townley S, Amanfo L, Henderson CR, et al. Preparing to implement a self-management program for back pain in New York city senior centers: what do prospective customers think? Pain Med. 2010;11:405–15.
47. Austrian J, Kerns RD, Reid MC. Perceived barriers to the use of self-management strategies for chronic pain in older persons. J Am Geriatr Soc. 2005;53:856–61.
48. Christo PJ, Li S, Gibson SJ, et al. Effective treatments for pain in the older patient. Curr Pain Headache Rep. 2011;15:22–34.
49. Brady TJ, Jernick SL, Hootman JM, Sniezek JE. Public health interventions for arthritis: expanding the toolbox of evidence-based interventions. J Women's Health. 2009;18:1905–17.
50. Arthritis-Foundation. Arthritis foundation self-help program safe and effective: outcomes summary. Available from: http://www.arthritis.org/media/programs/Evaluation_Summary_SelfHelp_HIGH.pdf.
51. Lorig K, Lubeck D, Kraines RG, Seleznick M, Holman HR. Outcomes of self-help education for patients with arthritis. Arthritis Rheum. 1985;28:680–5.
52. Hirano PC, Laurent DD, Lorig K. Arthritis patient education studies, 1987–1991: a review of the literature. Patient Educ Couns. 1994;24:9–54.
53. Brady TJ, Kruger J, Helmick CG, Callahan LF, Boutaugh ML. Intervention programs for arthritis and other rheumatic diseases. Health Educ Behav. 2003;30:44–63.

54. Larson AM, Polson J, Fontana RJ, Davern TJ, Lalani E, et al. Acetaminophen-induced acute liver failure: results of a United States multicenter, prospective study. Hepatology. 2005;42(6):1364–72.
55. Laine L. Approaches to nonsteroidal anti-inflammatory drug use in the high-risk patient. Gastroenterology. 2001;120(3):594–606.
56. Talley NJ, Evan JM, Fleming KC, Harmsen WS, Zinsmeister AR, Melton LJ. Nonsteroidal anti-inflammatory drugs and dyspepsia in the elderly. Dig Dis Sci. 1995;40(6):1345–50.
57. Trelle S, Reichenbach S, Wandel S, et al. Cardiovascular safety of non-steroidal anti-inflammatory drugs: network meta-analysis. BMJ. 2011;342:c7086.
58. Reid MC, Papaleontiou M, Amanfo L, Olkhovskaya Y, Moore AA, Turner BJ. Use of opioids for chronic pain in older adults: treatment practices and outcomes. Pain Med. 2010;11:1063–71.
59. Solomon DH, Rassen JA, Glynn RJ, Lee J, Levin R, Schneeweiss S. The comparative safety of analgesics in older adults with arthritis. Arch Intern Med. 2010;170(22):1968–78.
60. Chou R, Haegerich TM, Dowell D. CDC guideline for prescribing opioids for chronic pain- United States, 2016. JAMA. 2016;315(15):1624–45.
61. Bellamy N, Campbell J, Robinson V, Gee T, Bourne R, Well G. Viscosupplementation for the treatment of osteoarthritis of the knee. Cochrane Database Syst Rev. 2005;(1):CD005321.

Pain Assessment in Older Adults

Abisola B. Mesioye and Grace A. Cordts

Pain is a common symptom in older adults as detailed in the chapter "Effective Approaches for Pain Relief in Older Adults". Although common, it is underrecognized and undertreated in the elderly. This inadequate recognition and treatment leads to depression, social isolation, immobility, sleep disturbance, and decrease in quality of life for older persons [1, 2]. Thus, it is important for providers to recognize pain and treat it in the elderly to prevent increased morbidity. An effective pain management approach generally includes assessment and treatment steps outlined in Table 1. This chapter will focus on pain assessment with an overview of implications for management.

This basic approach to pain management is similar regardless of age, but there are challenges to pain management in the elderly, especially as sensory and cognitive impairments worsen and comorbidities occur. Table 2 lists some of these challenges. Multiple chronic diseases place the elderly at high risk for poor quality of life, physical disability, high health-care costs, adverse drug events, and mortality. The clinician caring for an elderly person with multiple comorbidities needs to consider patient preferences, the available evidence, prognosis, and clinical feasibility in deciding how to approach pain issues [3, 4]. The caregiver is an important source of information in the assessment and is integral in the implementation of a care plan when a patient has increasing cognitive and sensory impairments. This is especially important because over half (55.1%) of older adults in noninstitutionalized settings lived with their spouse, while 29% lived alone, according to a 2010 survey [5]. It is important to evaluate caregiver burden since a caregiver can be integral to a pain

---

A. B. Mesioye (✉)
Geriatrics and Extended Care Clinical Center, VA Maryland Health Care System,
Perry Point, MD, USA

Department of Medicine, University of Maryland School of Medicine, Baltimore, MD, USA
e-mail: Abisola.mesioye@va.gov

G. A. Cordts
Optum, Complex Care Management, Pittsburgh, PA, USA

© Springer Science+Business Media, LLC, part of Springer Nature 2019
G. A. Cordts, P. J. Christo (eds.), *Effective Treatments for Pain in the Older Patient*,
https://doi.org/10.1007/978-1-4939-8827-3_2

Table 1 Common approach to pain management

1. Assessment
(a) History
(i) Description of pain
1. Onset
2. Duration
3. Associated symptoms
4. Aggravating/relieving factors
5. Treatments and medications tried and response
(ii) Past medical history
(iii) Medications
(iv) Caregiver assessment (if applicable)
(v) Functional assessment
(vi) Cognitive assessment
(vii) Emotional assessment
(b) Physical exam
(c) Appropriate studies
2. Treatment
(a) Treatment guided by patient preference, goals of care
(b) Treat underlying causes found if appropriate
(c) Nonpharmacological and pharmacological approaches

Table 2 Challenges of pain assessment in the elderly

Elderly patient acceptance of pain as a normal part of aging leading to underreporting
Sensory and cognitive impairments
Comorbidities complicating the clinical picture
Provider's belief that if the person does not complain of pain, there is no pain
Fears of addiction on the part of the patient and provider
Difference in assessment of pain on the part of person, caregiver, and provider
Lack of good evidence to make informed treatment decisions
Elderly patients often presenting atypically
More than one type of pain occurring at one time

management plan. For instance, if a caregiver is overwhelmed, they might find it difficult to bring their loved one to multiple physical therapy sessions or remember to give medication several times during the day.

Pain assessment is the cornerstone of high-quality pain management. It is an ongoing process with an initial comprehensive assessment and ongoing reassessments for monitoring interventions. In the elderly, pain assessment is complex and involves many domains including physical, emotional, psychological, cognitive, and functional domains [6].

The purpose of the initial pain assessment is to:

1. Diagnose to determine the cause of pain
2. Identify comorbidities that impact the expression of pain such as dementia or depression

3. Identify effects on physical and emotional function from ongoing pain
4. Identify comorbidities that influence the choice of treatments such as dementia, congestive heart failure, renal failure, or hypertension
5. Identify factors that impact the treatment plan, such as caregiver stress or the specific living situation

The comprehensive pain assessment includes a good history, physical exam, and appropriate studies, with consideration given to patient preferences, life expectancy, and goals of care. The provider should ensure that patient has all assistive devices (e.g., eyeglasses, hearing aids) for all evaluations.

> **Clinical Scenario: Presentation**
> Mr. M is an 83-year-old community-dwelling elder, who presents in your clinic with chronic leg pain. He lives with his wife of 50 years, who is also his primary caregiver. He has a PMH of CHF, DM, and dementia. His medications include furosemide, glyburide, and aspirin. He is able to answer some questions but cannot give an adequate history. His wife states he started getting up at night and falling 1 month ago and has fallen four times with no injury. He comes to the office because he could not get up by himself.

History

The history includes a description of pain, medications used for pain (prescription and over-the-counter medications), the effectiveness and side effects of medications used, nonpharmacologic treatments used for pain management, assessment of comorbidities, and assessment of functional status, cognitive status, emotional status, and caregiver stress. Attitudes about pain and pain management can influence the willingness to try different approaches to pain management and thus need to be discussed. For example, if a patient or family member is concerned about addiction with opioids, they may not adhere to a medication treatment plan that includes opioids.

Description of Pain

Self-report is the gold standard for determining if pain is present. There is no test to say whether or not a person has pain. People with chronic pain do not have the autonomic indicators of acute pain such as tachycardia or hypertension, so providers often do not think someone is in pain if they look comfortable. This creates a barrier to good pain management. Elderly often do not report pain and need to be asked about it.

A detailed pain history includes the location of the pain, its duration, character, intensity, temporal patterns, radiating features, precipitating factors, aggravating factors, and relieving factors. A pain diary may be a good source of information. This is a simple record with a description of the pain each time it occurred over several days or weeks [7]. When asking about pain, it is important to use other descriptors of pain such as aching or hurting since some older patients will deny pain but acknowledge other descriptors of pain [6]. Intensity of pain is important to assess. It gives a benchmark for evaluating effectiveness of treatment. Although the intensity of pain is subjective, it is a benchmark that can be used to see if treatment has been effective. The intensity of pain is assessed using one of many unidimensional or multidimensional scales available. Unidimensional scales are single item scales about pain intensity. They are easy to administer with little training and give valid and reliable results. They do require good vision, hearing, and attention as well as the use of pencil and paper for some of the scales. Figure 1 shows examples of these types of scales, such as numeric rating scales, graphic picture scales, word descriptor scales, and visual analogue scales. Visual analogue scales have been shown in some studies to be more difficult for older adults to use, so they should be avoided [8].

Multidimensional tools take into account other factors such as the sensory quality and affective contributions to the pain. These tools are often impractical in the clinical setting due to their complexity and the length of time required to administer them. The short-form McGill Pain Questionnaire [9] is a multidimensional scale that has been shown to be consistent, reliable, and fairly easy to use. The same scale should be used at each reassessment to standardize the evaluation and to help with assessing the effectiveness of treatment.

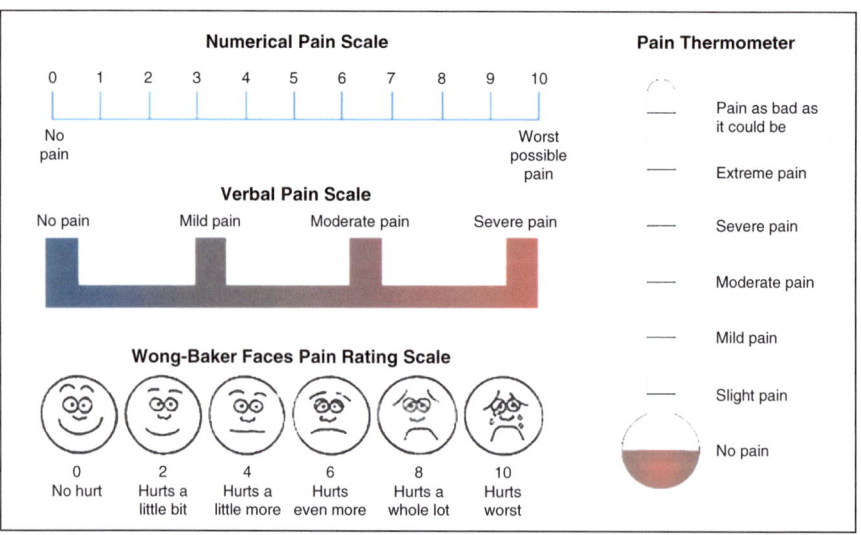

Fig. 1 Wong-Baker FACES Pain Rating Scale with permission from Wong-Baker FACES Foundation. (Pain thermometer with permission from Herr and Mobily [35])

People with advanced dementia and people with no verbal abilities often cannot express that they have pain. They can present with functional decline or behavioral issues such as agitation and aggression. The practitioner needs to keep this in mind when a functional decline occurs or someone has a new or exacerbated behavioral issue. In these cases, self-report may not be an option, and they cannot use the scales traditionally used in pain assessment. It is suggested to proceed with a hierarchy of assessments for nonverbal patients as outlined in Table 3. Often a combination of these approaches is needed to assess pain in these patients. Attempts should be made to obtain the patient's self-report of pain, and interview the patient's caregiver in conjunction with observing and recording nonverbal pain indicators. It is important to keep in mind that surrogate assessments of pain are not always accurate. Caregivers tend to overestimate pain intensity and health-care providers underestimate pain [10, 11]. Caregivers can be coached to be more accurate in their assessment of pain [12]. If an elderly person has a condition that typically causes pain, it is reasonable to treat for pain. If an objective cause of pain is not found, an analgesic trial may be warranted and the patient closely monitored. One study shows that treating demented patients with analgesics significantly improves agitation, overall neuropsychiatric symptoms, and pain [13].

The American Geriatrics Society (AGS) and American Medical Directors Association (AMDA) consider behavioral observation-based assessment of pain best practice. Table 4 shows a list of common pain behaviors in cognitively impaired older adults developed by the AGS [14].

There are several behavioral assessment scales available in the literature. Examples of these behavioral scales can be found at http://prc.coh.org/pain-noa.htm. Two examples of behavioral scales are the Pain Assessment in Advanced Dementia (PAINAD) and the Checklist of Nonverbal Pain Indicators (CNPI).

The PAINAD scale is a behavior-observation tool developed for use in demented patients who cannot adequately verbalize pain [15]. There are five specific indicators on the scale: breathing, vocalization, facial expression, body language, and consolability (https://www.healthcare.uiowa.edu/igec/tools/pain/PAINAD.pdf). The CNPI is another behavior pain tool that is reliable and easy to use (https://www.healthcare.uiowa.edu/igec/tools/pain/nonverbalPain.pdf). A behavioral scale is completed with activity. The score does not indicate severity of pain as in the other tools of pain intensity. It indicates merely that pain may be present. The "score" can be helpful in evaluating treatment interventions over time. Additional discussions of pain assessment in patients not able to communicate are found in chapter "A Biopsychosocial Perspective on the Assessment and Treatment of Chronic Pain in Older Adults".

Table 3 Hierarchy of assessment

1. Self-report
2. Search for potential causes
3. Observe patient behaviors
4. Proxy reports
5. Attempt an analgesic trial

Adapted from Herr et al. [33]

Table 4 Common pain behaviors in cognitively impaired elderly persons

Facial expressions
Slight frown; sad, frightened face
Grimacing, wrinkled forehead, closed or tightened eyes
Any distorted expression
Rapid blinking
Verbalizations, vocalizations
Sighing, moaning, groaning
Grunting, chanting, calling out
Noisy breathing
Asking for help
Verbally abusive
Body movements
Rigid, tense body posture, guarding
Fidgeting
Increased pacing, rocking
Restricted movement
Gait or mobility changes
Changes in interpersonal interactions
Aggressive, combative, resisting care
Decreased social interactions
Socially inappropriate, disruptive
Withdrawn
Changes in activity patters or routines
Refusing food, appetite change
Increase in rest periods
Sleep, rest pattern changes
Sudden cessation of common routines
Increased wandering
Mental status changes
Crying or tears
Increased confusion
Irritability or distress

Source: AGS Panel on Persistent Pain in Older Persons [14]. Used with permission
Note: Some patients demonstrate little or no specific behavior associated with severe pain

Past Medical History (PMH)

The goal of reviewing the PMH is to identify conditions that influence pain perception and behavior, to identify possible sources of pain, and to identify conditions that influence treatment.

Cognitive impairment, mood disorders, cerebrovascular disease, and degenerative neurological disorders are conditions that influence pain perception and behavior. There are many conditions that can cause acute and chronic pain in the elderly. Table 5 lists common diseases causing pain. Renal disease and liver failure influence the medication choice for pain treatment. Current or past alcohol or other illicit drug use is an important part of the history. If the patient is living at home, a home

Table 5 Common diseases causing pain

Somatic/MSK
Spinal stenosis – cervical, lumbar
Poor positioning in bedbound
PMR/DJD/RA/gout
Occult fracture, failure of old prosthetics
Osteoporosis/compression fractures
Contractures
Pressure sores
Oral/dental lesions
Paget's disease
Neuropathic
Poststroke pain
Claudication/PVD
Peripheral neuropathy – diabetic, phantom
Shingles/postherpetic
Trigeminal neuralgia
Drug-induced (chemo, EtoH)
Visceral
Mesenteric ischemia
Cancer

safety assessment is helpful. There are many checklists found on the Internet. One such is found at http://www.unmc.edu/homeinsteadcenter/docs/Home_Safety_Checklist-11.pdf.

Medications

Medication review includes all medications including over-the-counter medications. It is suggested elderly patients bring all their medications with them to outpatient visits, including all over-the-counter medications. Often patients who are in pain take over-the-counter medications. Elderly patients are at greater risk for drug interactions and drug side effects. It is not uncommon to find these patients taking several types of similar over-the-counter medications. For example, they may be taking both naproxen and ibuprofen. Commercials on television can be very enticing, and people do not realize that these medications are from the same drug class. They may be taking a combination pain medication, which includes an opioid and acetaminophen, and taking over-the-counter acetaminophen exposing them to potential overdose of acetaminophen. The total dose of acetaminophen should not exceed 3–4 grams of acetaminophen daily. Medications need to be reviewed for strength, dose route, frequency, actual use of the medications, effect on pain, adverse reactions, and length of medication use.

Other factors may affect medication use. If a patient has had a side effect from a medication, they might be unwilling to try it again. Also, cost can be an important consideration, so be sure to inquire about the patient's prescription medicine plan. This can effect what medications a patient is able to obtain.

Caregiver Assessment (if Applicable)

The caregiver is an important source of information particularly when the care recipient is an elderly patients with advanced dementia. A caregiver's assessment of the patient's pain can supplement self-description.

Alternately, caregivers can be burdened themselves due to the physical, emotional, and financial stress associated with caring for their loved ones. Consequently, pain assessment of a patient includes an evaluation of caregiver stress. This is particularly important as the caregiver's role is crucial for the implementation of the care plan [16]. Methods of relieving caregiver stress are included in the plan of care if indicated. Caregiver stress can be evaluated by simply asking the caregiver about stress or selecting from a wide variety of clinical tools [17]. These include the Zarit Burden Scale (Table 6) [18] and the American Medical Association's Caregiver Self-assessment Questionnaire (Table 7).

Table 6 The Zarit Burden interview: short version and screening version*

	Do you feel…	Never	Rarely	Sometimes	Quite frequently	Nearly always
*2	That because of the time you spend with your relative, you don't have enough time for yourself?	0	1	2	3	4
*3	Stressed between caring for your relative and trying to meet other responsibilities (work/family)?	0	1	2	3	4
5	Angry when you are around your relative?	0	1	2	3	4
6	That your relative currently affects your relationship with family members or friends in a negative way?	0	1	2	3	4
*9	Strained when you are around your relative?	0	1	2	3	4
10	That your health has suffered because of your involvement with your relative?	0	1	2	3	4
11	That you don't have as much privacy as you would like because of your relative?	0	1	2	3	4
12	That your social life has suffered because you are caring for your relative?	0	1	2	3	4
17	That you have lost control of your life since your relative's illness?	0	1	2	3	4
*19	Uncertain what to do about your relative?	0	1	2	3	4
20	You should be doing more for your relative?	0	1	2	3	4
21	You could do a better job in caring for your relative?	0	1	2	3	4

Used with permission, Oxford University Press. Bedard et al. [18]

Table 7 Caregiver self-assessment questionnaire. Permission courtesy of Health in Aging (this questionnaire was originally developed and tested by the American Medical Association)

Caregivers are often so concerned with caring for the relative's needs that they lose sight of their own well-being. Please take just a moment to answer the following questions. Once you have answered the questions, please also complete the self-evaluation

Answering "Yes" or "No" to the following questions, during the past week or so, I have…

1. Had trouble keeping my mind on what I was doing
2. Felt that I couldn't leave my relative alone
3. Had difficulty making decisions
4. Felt completely overwhelmed
5. Felt lonely
6. Been upset that my relative has changed so much from his/her former self
7. Felt a loss of privacy and/or personal time
8. Been edgy or irritable
9. Had sleep disturbed because of caring for my relative
10. Had a crying spell(s)
11. Felt strained between work and family responsibilities
12. Had back pain
13. Felt ill (*headaches, stomach problems, or common cold*)
14. Been satisfied with the support my family has given me
15. Found my relative's living situation to be inconvenient or a barrier to care
16. On a scale of 1 to 10, with 1 being "not stressful" to 10 being "extremely stressful," please rate your current level of stress
17. On a scale of 1 to 10, with 1 being "very healthy" to 10 being "very ill," please rate your current health compared to what it was this time last year

Self-evaluation

To determine the score

1. Reverse score questions 5 and 14. *For example, a "No" response should be counted as a "Yes" and a "Yes" response should be counted as a "No"*
2. Total the number of "Yes" responses

To interpret the score

Chances are that you are experiencing a high degree of distress if any of the below is true

If you answered "Yes" to either or both questions 4 and 10
If your total "Yes" scores = 9 or more
If your score on question 16 is 6 or higher
If your score on question 17 is 6 or higher

Next steps

Consider seeing a doctor for a checkup for yourself
Consider having some relief from caregiving
Discuss with your health-care provider or a social worker the resources available in your community
Consider joining a support group

Valuable resources for caregivers

HealthinAging.org
(800) 563–4916
www.healthinaging.org

(continued)

Table 7 (continued)

Eldercare Locator (*a national directory of community services*) (800) 677–1116 www.eldercare.gov	
Family Caregiver Alliance (800) 445–8106 www.caregiver.org	
Medicare hotline (800) 633–4227 www.medicare.gov	
National Alliance for Caregiving (301) 718–8444 www.caregiving.org	

Functional Assessment

Assessing functional status is important. There is a wide variation in function for elderly patients of the same age, directly affecting their life expectancies and goals of care. Functional status is affected by pain. Consequently the improvement in functional status is often a goal of pain management. Furthermore, the effect of pain on function can be an indicator of pain severity. Hence, function can be useful for monitoring treatment response. Function can be evaluated by asking about the elder's ability to perform the basic tasks of everyday life, also known as the activities of daily living (ADLS) and instrumental activities of daily living (IADLS). An example of a scale for ADLS can be found at http://consultgerirn.org/uploads/File/trythis/try_this_2.pdf. Table 8 is an example of a scale for IADLS [19]. A detailed discussion of functional assessment in patients with chronic pain is found in chapter "A Biopsychosocial Perspective on the Assessment and Treatment of Chronic Pain in Older Adults".

Cognitive Assessment

Cognitive impairment can impact the perception of pain, can be worsened by pain, and is a risk factor for delirium. Therefore all older adults should have a cognitive screen, such as the Mini- Cog (http://www.alz.org/documents_custom/minicog.pdf), which is a simple 3-min screening test. An abnormal screen should prompt more detailed neuropsychological testing if indicated. The results will be useful when deciding which pain assessment tools should be used, as patients with dementia may need specialized pain scales as discussed earlier.

Many elderly are at high risk for delirium on the account of age, multiple comorbidities, cognitive and visual impairment, and functional impairment [20]. Delirium is assessed for at the initial interview. Delirium is an acute confusional state that is diagnosed based on a history of acute change and fluctuation in mental status, inattention, disorganized thinking, and altered level of consciousness [20]. These features can be assessed using the Confusion Assessment Method (CAM), a clinical

Table 8 Instrumental activities of daily living (IADL)

A. Ability to use the telephone	
1. Operates telephone on own initiative; looks up and dials numbers, etc. (1)	
2. Dials a few well-known numbers (1)	
3. Answers telephone but does not dial (1)	
4. Does not use telephone at all (0)	
B. Shopping	
1. Takes care of all shopping needs independently (1)	
2. Shops independently for small purchases (0)	
3. Needs to be accompanied on any shopping trip (0)	
4. Completely unable to shop (0)	
C. Food preparation	
1. Plans, prepares, and serves adequate meals independently (1)	
2. Prepares adequate meals if supplied with ingredients (0)	
3. Heats, serves, and prepares meals or prepares meals but does not maintain adequate diet (0)	
4. Needs to have meals prepared and served (0)	
D. Housekeeping	
1. Maintains house alone or with occasional assistance (e.g., "heavy work domestic help") (1)	
2. Performs light daily tasks such as dishwashing, bed making (1)	
3. Performs light daily tasks but cannot maintain acceptable level of cleanliness (1)	
4. Needs help with all home maintenance tasks (1)	
5. Does not participate in any housekeeping tasks (0)	
E. Laundry	
1. Does personal laundry completely (1)	
2. Launders small items; rinses stockings, etc. (1)	
3. All laundry must be done by others (0)	
F. Mode of transportation	
1. Travels independently on public transportation or drives own car (1)	
2. Arranges own travel via taxi, but does not otherwise use public transportation (1)	
3. Travels on public transportation when accompanied by another (1)	
4. Travel limited to taxi or automobile with assistance of another (0)	
5. Does not travel at all (0)	
G. Responsibility for own medications	
1. Is responsible for taking medication in correct dosages at correct time (1)	
2. Takes responsibility if medication is prepared in advance in separate dosage (0)	
3. Is not capable of dispensing own medication (0)	
H. Ability to handle finances	
1. Manages financial matters independently (budgets, writes checks, pays rent, bills go to bank), collects and keeps track of income (1)	
2. Manages day-to-day purchases but needs help with banking, major purchases, etc. (1)	
3. Incapable of handling money (0)	

From Lawton and Brody [19]. Permission courtesy of the Gerontological Society of America, with permission of the Publisher tool used to establish the diagnosis of delirium (http://www.hospitalelderlifeprogram.org/delirium-instruments/short-cam/). The presence of delirium is associated with poor patient outcomes. Efforts to prevent it should be undertaken in all elderly patients with risk factors. Poorly controlled pain has been associated with delirium, while certain pain medications can cause delirium.

Emotional Assessment

Depression contributes to the severity of the pain and is a response to untreated pain. Two well-validated scales for diagnosing depression in older adults are the Geriatric Depression Scale (Table 9) [21] and the Patient Health Questionnaire Depression Scale (Table 10). See chapter "A Biopsychosocial Perspective on the Assessment and Treatment of Chronic Pain in Older Adults" for a detailed discussion of depression and pain.

Physical Exam

The physical examination is detailed and includes a focused musculoskeletal, vascular, and neurological exam, as these disorders frequently cause persistent pain in the elderly [22]. Persistent pain is defined as a painful experience that continues for a prolonged period of time, which may or may not be associated with a recognizable disease process [13]. The absence of findings does not mean pain is not present. Knowledge of the normal changes in aging is important so that normal changes are not misinterpreted as a cause of pain.

Pain is a factor in falls and diminished mobility in the elderly [23]. Gait and balance should be evaluated. The timed "up and go" test is a clinically useful measure of gait and mobility [24].

Appropriate Studies

The results of the history and physical might indicate further workup to determine the etiology of pain. The amount of additional workup is dependent on the patient's current situation, life expectancy, goals of care, and patient/family preference. For example, further workup is probably not required for the evaluation of an elderly person on hospice but considered appropriate for evaluating an elderly person with a reasonable life expectancy. Any test ordered should have the goal of informing the treatment plan.

Vitamin D deficiency has been associated with pain, although the data are conflicting [25, 26]. Frail institutionalized elderly are at risk for vitamin D deficiency, so screening for vitamin D deficiency is appropriate. Replete vitamin D if deficiency is found. This is easy to do, may impact other conditions, and could make a difference by improving the pain.

Table 9 Geriatric Depression Scale (Long Form). Instructions: Choose the best answer for how you felt over the past week

No.	Question	Answer	Score
1.	Are you basically satisfied with your life?	Yes/no	
2.	Have you dropped many of your activities and interests?	Yes/no	
3.	Do you feel that your life is empty?	Yes/no	
4.	Do you often get bored?	Yes/no	
5.	Are you hopeful about the future?	Yes/no	
6.	Are you bothered by thoughts you can't get out of your head?	Yes/no	
7.	Are you in good spirits most of the time?	Yes/no	
8.	Are you afraid that something bad is going to happen to you?	Yes/no	
9.	Do you feel happy most of the time?	Yes/no	
10.	Do you often feel helpless?	Yes/no	
11.	Do you often get restless and fidgety?	Yes/no	
12.	Do you prefer to stay at home, rather than going out and doing new things?	Yes/no	
13.	Do you frequently worry about the future?	Yes/no	
14.	Do you feel you have more problems with memory than most?	Yes/no	
15.	Do you think it is wonderful to be alive now?	Yes/no	
16.	Do you often feel downhearted and blue?	Yes/no	
17.	Do you feel pretty worthless the way you are now?	Yes/no	
18.	Do you worry a lot about the past?	Yes/no	
19.	Do you find life very exciting?	Yes/no	
20.	Is it hard for you to get started on new projects?	Yes/no	
21.	Do you feel full of energy?	Yes/no	
22.	Do you feel that your situation is hopeless?	Yes/no	
23.	Do you feel that most people are better off than you are?	Yes/no	
24.	Do you frequently get upset over little things?	Yes/no	
25.	Do you frequently feel like crying?	Yes/no	
26.	Do you have trouble concentrating?	Yes/no	
27.	Do you enjoy getting up in the morning?	Yes/no	
28.	Do you prefer to avoid social gatherings?	Yes/no	
29.	Is it easy for you to make decisions?	Yes/no	
30.	Is your mind as clear as it used to be?	Yes/no	
Total			

From Yesavage et al. [21]. Used with permission of Oxford University Press
This is the original scoring for the scale: one point for each of these answers
Cutoff: normal, 0–9; mild depressive, 10–19; severe depressives, 20–30

1. No	6. Yes	11. Yes	16. Yes	21. No	26. Yes
2. Yes	7. No	12. Yes	17. Yes	22. Yes	27. No
3. Yes	8. Yes	13. Yes	18. Yes	23. Yes	28. Yes
4. Yes	9. No	14. Yes	19. No	24. Yes	29. No
5. No	10. Yes	15. No	20. Yes	25. Yes	30. No

Table 10 Patient Health Questionnaire (PHQ-9). Over the last 2 weeks; how often have you been bothered by any of the following problems?

PATIENT HEALTH QUESTIONNAIRE (PHQ-9)

NAME:_____   DATE:_____

Over the last *2 weeks,* how often have you been bothered by any of the following problems?
(use "✓" to indicate your answer)

	Not at all	Several days	More than half the days	Nearly every day
1. Little interest or pleasure in doing things	0	1	2	3
2. Feeling down, depressed, or hopeless	0	1	2	3
3. Trouble falling or staying asleep, or sleeping too much	0	1	2	3
4. Feeling tired or having little energy	0	1	2	3
5. Poor appetite or overeating	0	1	2	3
6. Feeling bad about yourself—or that you are a failure or have let yourself or your family down	0	1	2	3
7. Trouble concentrating on things, such as reading the newspaper or watching television	0	1	2	3
8. Moving or speaking so slowly that other people could have noticed. Or the opposite — being so figety or restless that you have been moving around a lot more than usual	0	1	2	3
9. Thoughts that you would be better off dead, or of hurting yourself	0	1	2	3

add columns   _____ + _____ + _____

(Healthcare professional: For interpretation of TOTAL, please refer to accompanying scoring card).   TOTAL: _____

10. If you checked off *any problems,* how *difficult* have these problems made it for you to do your work, take care of things at home, or get along with other people?	Not difficult at all _____ Somewhat difficult _____ Very difficult _____ Extremely difficult _____

Copyright © 1999 Pfizer inc. All rights reserved. Reproduced with permission. PRIME-MD© is a trademark of Pfizer Inc.
A2663B 10-04-2005

Table 10 (continued)

PHQ-9 Patient Depression Questionnaire

For initial diagnosis:

1. Patient completes PHQ-9 Quick Depression Assessment.
2. If there are at least 4 ✓s in the shaded section (including Questions #1 and #2), consider a depressive disorder. Add score to determine severity.

Consider Major Depressive Disorder
 - if there are at least 5 ✓s in the shaded section (one of which corresponds to Question #1 or #2)

Consider Other Depressive Disorder
 - if there are 2-4 ✓s in the shaded section (one of which corresponds to Question #1 or #2)

Note: Since the questionnaire relies on patient self-report, all responses should be verified by the clinician, and a definitive diagnosis is made on clinical grounds taking into account how well the patient understood the questionnaire, as well as other relevant information from the patient.
Diagnoses of Major Depressive Disorder or Other Depressive Disorder also require impairment of social, occupational, or other important areas of functioning (Question #10) and ruling out normal bereavement, a history of a Manic Episode (Bipolar Disorder), and a physical disorder, medication, or other drug as the biological cause of the depressive symptoms.

To monitor severity over time for newly diagnosed patients or patients in current treatment for depression:

1. Patients may complete questionnaires at baseline and at regular intervals (eg, every 2 weeks) at home and bring them in at their next appointment for scoring or they may complete the questionnaire during each scheduled appointment.
2. Add up ✓s by column. For every ✓: Several days = 1 More than half the days = 2 Nearly every day = 3
3. Add together column scores to get a TOTAL score.
4. Refer to the accompanying **PHQ-9 Scoring Box** to interpret the TOTAL score.
5. Results may be included in patient files to assist you in setting up a treatment goal, determining degree of response, as well as guiding treatment intervention.

Scoring: add up all checked boxes on PHQ-9

For every ✓ Not at all = 0; Several days = 1;
More than half the days = 2; Nearly every day = 3

Interpretation of Total Score

Total Score	Depression Severity
1-4	Minimal depression
5-9	Mild depression
10-14	Moderate depression
15-19	Moderately severe depression
20-27	Severe depression

PHQ9 Copyright © Pfizer Inc. All rights reserved. Reproduced with permission. PRIME-MD ® is a trademark of Pfizer Inc.

A2662B 10-04-2005

Table 11 Red flags

Red flag	Possible causes
History of cancer Unexplained weight loss Loss of bladder and bowel Pain worse at night or when supine Significant acute sensory deficit or motor weakness	Cancer
Severe osteoporosis Minor or major trauma	Fracture
Fever Chills Night sweats Urinary tract infection Recent instrumentation	Infection

Red Flags

There are a few signs and symptoms from the initial history and physical referred to as red flags that can be indicators of serious underlying disease, including cancer, infection, and fracture [27]. See Table 11. These "red flags" were first described in low back pain but are applicable to any pain presentation. There is no single red flag, and many have false positives, which can add to cost and outcomes. Frail elderly are at risk of adverse outcomes from testing. Nevertheless providers should be aware of these and consider further workup if appropriate.

> **Clinical Scenario: Assessment**
> Mr. M can only tell you that his legs hurt all over. He cannot give any more history and gets agitated when you ask him further questions. He is also unable to quantify the pain using a number or identifying a face. His wife states that the patient has had pain in his legs since he retired 13 years ago, and they both felt this was normal for his age. She thinks he may be pointing to his right foot more often when she asks him where it hurts. She is not aware of aggravating or relieving factors but has noticed that Mr. M. spends more time in bed and will no longer take walks with her. He is combative when she tries to bathe and dress him, and she noticed that he winced when she was putting on his socks and shoes. The patient is dependent in all his instrumental activities of daily living and needs help with dressing and bathing. He was able to transfer independently until 2 days ago, which is the reason for the visit. He is still able to eat on his own, but his appetite has decreased. He fell a month ago. The patient had woken up at night to go to the bathroom, as was his usual habit, and his wife heard a loud thud in the bathroom. She found him sitting

on the floor but was able to get him back to bed. Since that episode he has complained of more pain in his legs and is now wearing an adult brief, as he can no longer get out of bed to go to the bathroom without assistance and has had a few episodes of functional incontinence. Review of the medical record shows that his last MMSE score was 18/30. The patient was able to complete the Geriatric Depression Scale assisted by his wife and scored 10/30 indicating mild depression. His PAINAD score is 5 indicating pain is present. When you interview Mrs. M, she states that she is exhausted and is considering nursing home placement. Her score on the Zarit Burden Scale is 64.

Mr. M is found to be a frail elder who looks tense and anxious. He grimaces from time to time. He talks in low tones with a disapproving quality. He seems to be reassured when you touch his shoulder. Pertinent physical examination findings include bilateral cataracts with visual acuity 20/60 in his left eye and 20/40 in his right eye. There are a few scattered crackles in both lower lobes on chest auscultation. Neurological exam shows bilateral impairment of pain, light touch, and temperature in a "stocking" pattern. There are also loss of vibratory sensation, altered proprioception, and absent ankle reflexes. He has good pulses in his feet. Power is 4/5 in both lower limbs. Mr. M. is unable to get up from a sitting position. After he is helped up, you notice that his gait is slow and very unsteady. He asks to sit down after a few steps.

You perform some lab tests and get X-rays of both feet. Significant lab findings include glycosylated hemoglobin level of 7.8, a random blood sugar of 250, an albumin level of 3.0, and blood urea nitrogen and creatinine of 30 and 1.5, respectively. The X-rays show mild degenerative joint disease and osteopenia.

The history and physical exam findings indicate that Mr. M. may be experiencing pain from diabetic neuropathy and arthritis. This has led to a significant functional decline. The unsteady gait and pain may have contributed to the fall as well as his poor visual acuity and cognitive impairment. His wife is experiencing severe caregiver stress.

Management Implications

The treatment plan is based on the working diagnosis from the assessment, the elderly person's unique combination of diseases and situation, their personal preferences, and the goals of treatment the patient and provider have agreed upon. The goals of intervention may include improvement in functional status, enhanced quality of life, increased comfort, improvement in sleep, or mitigation of pain-related mood disorders. The actual plan is usually multifaceted and includes nonpharmacologic and pharmacologic interventions deemed appropriate. The possible nonpharmacologic and pharmacologic interventions are discussed in subsequent chapters.

Of note, if an opioid is prescribed as part of the regimen, a clearly defined objective outcome for the use of the opioid should be defined related to both for pain and function. There should also be established criteria for stopping or continuing and reassessment of risks and benefits after initiating the treatment. The current opioid epidemic [28, 29] should not preclude the use of opioids for the management of moderate to severe pain in the elderly when the pain is not adequately relieved by nonpharmacologic methods and other pharmacologic agents.

The use of opioid medication is clearly related to adverse outcomes including overdose deaths, physical dependence, tolerance, sedation, delirium, constipation, and respiratory distress [30, 31]. However, organ toxicities are less common than with other analgesics such as nonsteroidal anti-inflammatory agents [32].

When opioid mediations are considered necessary for older adults, the starting dose should be lower than in younger adults and titrated up slowly with frequent assessment and reassessment of pain levels. The patient and caregiver should demonstrate understanding of the prescription instruction and potential side effects. In particular, such patients should be started on a bowel regimen and education given on monitoring for bowel movements.

A written plan of prescribed treatment is given to the patient and family. Close follow-up is arranged, and a plan on how to contact the provider is given for any questions or concerns that come up in the interim between visits.

Management of Pain in Nonverbal Patients or Patients with Advanced Dementia

Elderly with advanced dementia and the inability to communicate pain present not only an assessment challenge but also a management challenge. Often it is difficult to tell if a change in behavior or functional decline is related to pain. These behaviors and functional decline do not just indicate pain but can be any unmet need including physical (hunger, infection, pain, medication side effect), psychological (boredom, loneliness, lack of socialization), or psychiatric (depression, anxiety, delirium, psychosis) needs. Clinicians often must hypothesize about the etiology of the behavior and intervene based on the hypothesis and reassess for change in the behavior after the intervention. Table 12 suggests such an approach and is based on approach found on the following website: (https://www.healthcare.uiowa.edu/IGEC/IAAdapt/document/Problem_Behaviors_overall_approach_and_common_causes.pdf).

Documentation

Documentation of the initial assessment, treatment plan, and subsequent follow-up are necessary to communicate with other providers involved in the care of the patient. One format is outlined in Table 13. It is especially helpful if opioids are prescribed because it incorporates an evaluation of opioid misuse.

Table 12 Treatment strategy for elderly with severe dementia[a]

Step 1: A behavior is identified that might be pain
Step 2: Physical assessment/affective assessment; review of the recent history; environmental factors
Step 3: Trial of nonpharmacological comfort treatments
Step 4: Trial of analgesics
Step 5: If this does not work, consideration that pain is not the issue and reevaluation of the hypothesis
Proceed sequentially through these steps until the problem is treated and behavioral symptoms have returned to baseline or substantially improved.

[a]Adapted from the Iowa Geriatric Education Center https://www.healthcare.uiowa.edu/IGEC/IAAdapt/document/Problem_Behaviors_overall_approach_and_common_causes.pdf

Table 13 Six A's of treating pain

Analgesia (nonpharmacologic/pharmacologic)
Activities of daily living
Adverse effects
Aberrant drug behaviors
Assessment (treatment response)
Action plan (adjustments to treatment plan)

Adapted from Passik and Weinreb [34]

> **Clinical Scenario: Management and Follow-Up**
>
> Mr. M and his wife both state that they want him to remain at home for as long as possible. The goal is to improve his pain and functional status so he can remain at home. Mrs. M's caregiver burden needs to be addressed.
>
> You review the medical literature and explain the risks and benefits of the various pharmacologic agents for the management of diabetic neuropathy and osteoarthritis to Mrs. M, who is her husband's health-care agent. He is started on regular dosing of 650 mg of acetaminophen four times daily. His furosemide dose is changed to be administered every morning instead of every evening. He is also started on 300 mg of gabapentin every night and calcium and vitamin D supplements. Referrals are made for proper fitting diabetic footwear. Because Mr. M meets the definition of homebound, you make a referral to a Medicare-approved home health agency for physical therapy and evaluation of medications. The home health agency can provide a social worker and a home safety evaluation. You arrange follow-up in 2 weeks. Mrs. M. will contact you earlier if there is no significant improvement in the pain intensity and frequency. A plan of treatment is written down and provided to Mrs. M.
>
> At the follow-up visit, Mr. M is calmer, has had no falls, and no longer resists care. He is eating more and sleeping at night and no longer wakes up to go to the bathroom. He is receiving home PT, ambulates slowly with a cane,

and is wearing custom-made diabetic shoes. As a result of a home safety evaluation, scatter rugs by his bed have been removed, and grab bars have been installed in the bathroom. The home health agency also provides a home health aide, and Mrs. M is relieved of her caregiving responsibilities for 2 h a day.

Mr. M still complains of leg pain intermittently, and the decision is made to increase the gabapentin. Long-term goals are discussed with Mrs. M., who understands that her husband has moderate to severe dementia. She agrees to a referral to ophthalmology to evaluate his vision, establishing regular podiatry follow-up. Although Mr. M has diabetic neuropathy, the risk of hypoglycemia is thought to be greater than achieving tight diabetic control in view of his limited life expectancy, and his diabetic management is not changed.

Summary

Pain assessment and management in the elderly are important for the quality of life of elderly patients. The thorough assessment of pain involves many domains and the caregiver. It can be achieved by following the strategy outlined in this chapter.

- Undertreated pain leads to depression, social isolation, and loss of function.
- Pain assessment is the cornerstone of high-quality pain management.
- Reassessment of pain after intervention is important.
- The same assessment tools should be used to evaluate pain on each reevaluation.
- It is important to identify all the pain a patient has.
- Consider pain as an issue when behavioral and functional changes occur in elderly demented, nonverbal adults.
- Patients with advanced dementia or who are nonverbal need a hierarchical approach to pain assessment.
- Pain management is dependent on patient's goals, prognosis, and preferences.

References

1. Knott L. Treating osteoarthritis in practice—the TOP study. Curr Med Res Opin. 2000;16(2):147–52.
2. Kerns RD, Sellinger J, Goodin BR. Psychological treatment of chronic pain. Annu Rev Clin Psychol. 2011;7:411–34.
3. Boyd CM, et al. Clinical practice guidelines and quality of care for older patients with multiple comorbid diseases: implications for pay for performance. JAMA. 2005;294(6):716–24.
4. Guiding principles for the care of older adults with multimorbidity: an approach for clinicians. Guiding principles for the care of older adults with multimorbidity: an approach for clinicians: American Geriatrics Society Expert Panel on the care of older adults with multimorbidity. J Am Geriatr Soc. 2012;60(10):E1–E25.
5. A profile of older Americans: 2011 – Administration on aging, U.S. Department of Health and Human Services. Downloaded from http://www.aoa.gov/Aging_Statistics/Profile/2011/docs/2011profile.pdf.

6. Hadjistavropoulos T, et al. An interdisciplinary expert consensus statement on assessment of pain in older persons. Clin J Pain. 2007;23(1 Suppl):S1–S43.
7. Ferell BA. Pain management. In: Hazzard WR, editor. Principles of geriatric medicine and gerontology. 4th ed. New York: McGraw-Hill; 1998.
8. Gagliese L. Pain and aging: the emergence of a new subfield of pain research. J Pain. 2009;10(4):343–53.
9. Dworkin RH, Turk DC, Revicki DA, et al. Development and initial validation of an expanded and revised version of the short-form McGill pain questionnaire (SF-MPQ-2). Pain. 2009;144(1–2):35–42.
10. Herr K, Coyne PJ, Key T, et al. Pain assessment in the nonverbal patient: position statement with clinical practice recommendations. Pain Manag Nurs. 2006;7:44–51.
11. Puntillo K, Posino C, Li D, et al. Evaluation of pain in the ICU patients. Chest. 2009;135:1069–74.
12. Lobuchuk MM, Vorauer JD. Family caregiver perspective taking and accuracy in estimating cancer patient symptom experiences. Soc Sci Med. 2003;57:2379–84.
13. Husebo B, Ballard C, Sandvik R, et al. Efficacy of treating pain to reduce behavioral disturbances in residents of nursing homes with dementia: cluster randomized clinical trial. BMJ. 2011;343:d4065.
14. American Geriatric Society Panel on Persistent Pain in Older Persons. The management of persistent pain in older persons. J Am Geriatr Soc. 2002;50(6):S205–24.
15. Warden V, Hurley AC, Volicer L. Development and psychometric evaluation of the pain assessment in advanced dementia (PAINAD) scale. JAm Med Dir Assoc. 2003;4:9–15.
16. Gillick ME. The critical role of caregivers in achieving patient-centered care. JAMA. 2013;310(6):575–6.
17. Famakinwa A. Caregiver stress: the Physician's role. Geriatrics and Aging. 2009;12(5):267–9.
18. Bedard M, Molloy DW, Squire L, et al. The Zarit Burden Interview: a new short version and screening version. Gerontologist. 2001;41(5):652–7.
19. Lawton MP, Brody EM. Assessment of older people: self maintaining and instrumental activities of daily living. Gerontologist. 1969;9(3):179–86.
20. Inouye SK. Delirium in Older Persons. N Engl J Med. 2006;354:1157–65.
21. Yesavage JA, Brink TL, Rose TL, et al. Development and validation of a geriatric depression screening scale: a preliminary report. J Psychiatr Res. 1983;17(1):37–49.
22. American Geriatrics Society Panel on the Pharmacological Management of Persistent Pain in Older Persons. Pharmacological Management of Persistent Pain in Older Persons. J Am Geriatr Soc. 2009;57(8):1331–46.
23. Reid MC, Williams CS, Gill TM. Back pain and decline in lower extremity physical function among community-dwelling older persons. J Gerontol A Biol Sci Med Sci. 2005;60:793–7.
24. Podsiadlo D, Richardson S. The timed "Up and GO": a test of basic functional mobility for frail elderly persons. J Am Ger Soc. 1991;39:142–8.
25. Plotnikoff G, Quigley J. Prevalence of severe Hypoviaminosis D in patients with persistent, nonspecific musculoskeletal pain. Mayo Clin Proc. 2003;78(12):1463–70.
26. McAlindon T, LaValley M, Schneider E, et al. Effect of vitamin D supplementation on progression of knee pain and cartilage volume loss in patients with symptomatic osteoarthritis: a randomized control trial. JAMA. 2013;309:155–62.
27. Williams CM, Henschke N, Maher CG et al. Red Flags to screen for vertebral fracture in patients presenting with low back pain. Cochrane Database Syst Rev. 2013. https://doi.org/10.1002/14651858.CD008643.pub2. Published in the Cochran Library 2013 Issue 2.
28. Rudd RA, Aleshire N, Zibbel JE, et al. Increases in drug and opioid overdose deaths- United States, 2000–2014. MMWR. 2016;64(50):1378–82.
29. Dart RC, Surratt HL, Cicero TJ, et al. Trends in opioid analgesic abuse and mortality in the United States. N Engl J Med. 2015;372:2063–6.
30. Smith HS, King NB, Fraser V, Boikos C, et al. Determinants of increased opioid –related mortality in the United States and Canada, 1990-2013: a systemic review. Am J Public Health. 2014;104(8):e32–42. Opioid metabolism. Mayo Clin Proc. 2009;84 (7);613-62413.

31. Benyamin R, Trescott AM, Datta, et al. Opioid complications and side effects. Pain Physician. 2008;11(2 suppl):S105–20.
32. Marcum AZ, Hanlon JT. Recognizing the risks of chronic nonsteroidal anti-inflammatory drug use in older adults. Ann Longterm Care. 2010;18(9):24–7.
33. Herr K, Coyne P, McCaffery M, Manworren R, Merkel S. Pain assessment in patients unable to self-report: position statement with clinical practice recommendations. Pain Manag Nurs. 2011;12:230–50.
34. Passik SD, Weinreb HJ. Managing chronic nonmalignant pain: overcoming obstacles to the use of opioids. Adv Ther. 2000;17(2):70–83.
35. Herr KA, Mobily PR. Comparison of selected pain assessment tools for use with the elderly. Appl Nurs Res. 1993;6(11):39–46.

Acute Pain Management in Older Adults

Richard J. Lin and Eugenia L. Siegler

Prevalence and Impact of Acute Pain in Institutionalized Older Adults

Acute pain and acute exacerbation of chronic pain are highly prevalent in hospitalized patients across all settings, ranging from 37.7% to 84% for all pain quality and 9–36% for severe pain in a recent systemic review [1]. This kind of pain is especially prevalent among those admitted for surgery or cancer [2, 3] but also very common among general medical inpatients with more than 50% experiencing significant amounts of pain during their hospitalization [4, 5]. Moreover, there appears to be important variation in the quality of pain assessment and treatment for hospitalized patients, especially older adults [1–5].

It has been 40 years since the publication of a landmark study at two New York hospitals where nearly three-quarters of patients were in moderate or severe distress from pain [6]. Inpatient pain management has since improved slowly, and the Joint Commission's (TJC) first pain quality indicator was published in 2000 with the establishment of pain as the "fifth vital sign" [7]. Additional components deemed essential by TJC now include assessment that is tailored to the patient's age, condition, and comprehension, timely treatment, and timely reassessment. TJC has stated clearly and unequivocally that appropriate pain management is a patient right (PC.01.02.07).

Pain has been defined in the first chapters of this book. Acute pain is usually associated with tissue injury and has a temporal relationship with its onset and disappearance. It is commonly associated with objective physical signs of increased

R. J. Lin
Department of Medicine, Memorial Sloan Kettering Cancer Center, New York, NY, USA

E. L. Siegler (✉)
Division of Geriatrics and Palliative Medicine, Weill Cornell Medicine, New York, NY, USA
e-mail: els2006@med.cornell.edu

autonomic activity such as tachycardia, elevated blood pressure, diaphoresis, or anxiety. The neurologic basis of pain involves activation of peripheral and central pain pathways and can involve both normal and maladaptive physiological processes [8]. To understand the experience of acute pain in an institutionalized older patient, it is worth contemplating Dame Cicely Saunders' concept of total pain and its four domains of pain experience: physical, emotional, psychological, and social. She reminds us that these domains interact with each other and modulate each other's effects, while cultural factors and social context influence the expression and tolerance of pain [9]. The hospital and the circumstances that lead to hospitalization provide unique and important environmental and social contexts that influence the experience of pain and may complicate pain management. The disorientation caused by a recurrence of cancer, the sudden loss of function that attends a fracture, the emergency room, the loss of privacy, and threats to dignity can all be part of the experience of acute pain.

High-quality pain management in the acute setting remains a challenge. The negative consequences of poor inpatient pain management are substantial and include increased hospital costs (mostly driven by increased length of stay), as well as decreased patient satisfaction and quality of life [10]. Moreover, effective and timely management of acute pain is essential not only to relieve immediate suffering but also to prevent the development of chronic pain, which can result when unrelieved acute pain induces neuroplastic changes in pain pathways and central perceptions of pain [8]. Pain management in medical inpatients can be more complicated than in surgical patients, as they often have preexisting painful conditions such as arthritis, inflammatory diseases, cancer, or chronic neuropathic pain, as well as medical comorbidities that may preclude the use of specific analgesic medications.

Clinical Scenario
An 83-year-old woman was admitted for elective right total knee replacement. The surgery, which was uncomplicated, took place under general anesthesia and a local femoral nerve block. The patient was able to get out of bed to a chair the same afternoon and enjoy the company of her family. The next day, the pain worsened and the patient was given intramuscular (IM) morphine and several doses of intravenous (IV) hydromorphone, in addition to topical ice, standing celecoxib, and acetaminophen, with minimal relief. That evening, she became delirious and attempted to sit at the edge of the bed to improve her comfort. Worried for her safety, the nursing staff put her in a geri chair in the hallway until her family could arrive. She was able to sleep in the recliner and with a reduced dose of IV hydromorphone; there were no further episodes of delirium, although the patient complained of excessive fatigue and constipation. On day 4, the patient had not yet moved her bowels, despite docusate and senna. She was given milk of magnesia and then transferred to the rehabilitation unit. Several hours later, she developed cramping and became diaphoretic and hypotensive; placing her back in bed relieved these symptoms. She moved her bowels successfully

after an enema. The rest of her rehabilitation stay was uneventful, and she was an active participant in therapies when given IV hydromorphone as pretreatment and at bedtime. She was discharged home on oxycodone/APAP, where she completed her rehabilitation therapy and tapered off her opioids.

Comment: This case, elective surgery in a cognitively intact older woman without significant comorbidities, was nonetheless complicated by delirium, fatigue, constipation, and near syncope. Acute pain management is challenging in older patients under the best of circumstances, requiring frequent assessment, proper dosing, monitoring for relief and complications, and medication adjustment, but it is essential to successful recovery and rehabilitation, given the adverse long-term impact of poorly controlled acute pain.

Basic Assessment Tools in the Acute Setting

Pain assessment has been covered at length in chapter "Pain Assessment in Older Adults". There is a substantial literature on assessment tools in older patients and in those with cognitive impairment. In general, patients with even significant degrees of dementia can often give reliable verbal or numerical reports of pain. Chapter "Pain Assessment in Older Adults" also describes other tools that are available for staff use when the patient is nonverbal. These tools are often available on the patient care units and in documentation sections or flow sheets in the electronic health record (EHR). Our experience with demented patients who have acute pain, however, is that while they can report a level of pain when asked, they have difficulty placing pain in a context [11]. Table 1 lists some of the challenges of assessing pain in demented patients. Underlying dementia presents special difficulties when determining how to treat the pain because the emotional distress can be marked and intractable, interfering with rehabilitation and healing and at times causing great distress to the staff. Thus, while undertreatment of pain may occur due to inadequately assessed pain in demented patients, overtreatment may result from reflexively administering opioids and failing to help the patient contextualize the discomfort or to use modalities such as distraction to reduce the need for medication [12].

Table 1 Special challenges in demented patients

Lack of executive skills to recognize that a transfer may be painful but that once in the new position the pain will diminish or disappear
Failure to recognize that their pain score is lower and that pain has improved with treatment or time; and they may become frightened by pain that they think is new
Lack of response to verbal reassurance that they are improving because they may not believe it
Inability to recognize that the quality of pain has changed, leading clinicians to miss a postoperative or drug-induced complication

Acute Pain Management for Older Patients

Pain Management in the Emergency Department

Many hospitalizations for elderly begin in the emergency department (ED). More than 40% of ED visits for patients over 75 and more than half of elderly with fractures after falls are admitted to the hospital [13]. Even though definitive treatment is often left to the admitting team, pain should be treated promptly, starting in the ED. Treatment of acute pain in the ED does not differ substantially from inpatient units: it must be assessed, the appropriate medications must be prescribed and administered, and then the pain must be reassessed to ensure adequate analgesia. Nonetheless, depending on hospital policy, there may be some limitations in what is available to patients in the ED. Patient-controlled analgesia and standing opioid infusions (e.g., morphine drips), for example, may not be available if nursing staff have not been taught to manage PCA pumps.

Is pain treated differently in older than younger ED patients? Although earlier studies have suggested that older patients receive less medication or do not achieve pain relief [14, 15], a recent prospective study did not find "oligoanalgesia," and it is believed that factors such as patient preference, contraindications to opioid administration, better relief with disease-specific non-opioids, and poor chart abstraction may have compounded previous studies [16]. Older patients often desire to contribute to decisions regarding analgesics and should do so, but a recent prospective evaluation reveals that the shared decision-making does not necessarily lead to pain reduction [17]. Data do suggest that ED overcrowding leads not just to delays in assessment and treatment but in reassessment as well; in addition, the environment of the ED can worsen pain because of the noise, discomfort of gurneys, multiple procedures, and generalized stress of acute illness and uncertainty [15, 18].

The greatest challenge in pain management of patients admitted through the ED may be in the transition from ED to the floor. Transition times are dangerous under the best of circumstances; the handoff of an acutely ill patient from one team to another presents special challenges. None of these problems is specific to pain management, but all must be taken into account if the patient is to receive optimal care.

Unappreciated Medication Side Effects These complications may be in process even before the inpatient team takes responsibility. When the goal is to stabilize the patient, the adverse consequences of pain medications (constipation, delirium, renal impairment) may not be evident. Somnolence and delirium, in particular, may be attributed to a patient's underlying dementia when they in fact developed these symptoms after the patient arrived in the ED. Poor communication from shift to shift or between ED staff and inpatient staff about the patient's underlying cognitive and physical function can lead to continued inappropriate prescribing when no one is aware that the patient has deteriorated.

Suboptimal Handoffs A clinical provider may be admitting and managing multiple patients or handing off multiple patients at one time, and pain management may receive less attention than the diagnosis, treatment, and laboratory findings. The ED may be quite far away from the home unit of the accepting physician, slowing the response to pain; or pain management may not be discussed adequately during handoff due to perceived low priority.

EHR-Based Errors The ED may use a different EHR, or a unified hospital EHR may be programmed to treat the ED stay as separate from the inpatient admission; in many circumstances, it may be difficult to ascertain what medications the patient received and when. Patients who have been admitted but not yet assigned a bed may not receive the appropriate medications because orders written by the admitting team may not be active in the ED or may "fall off" upon the patient's transfer to an inpatient unit.

Recently, an important quality improvement (QI) project, Improving Pain Relief in Elder Patients (I-PREP), was carried out at the University of Chicago Medical Center [19]. This linked standardized education and continuous QI for multidisciplinary staff in the emergency department has led to significant reduction in pain severity, improved timing for pain assessment and reassessment, as well as faster delivery of pain medications to elderly patients with moderate-to-severe acute musculoskeletal and abdominal pain. This study suggests that the process of acute pain management can be standardized and improved using common QI technology.

Pain Management in the Hospital

Treating acute or acute on chronic pain in elderly can be challenging in the hospital setting [20, 21]. Older patients typically have more comorbidities than their younger counterparts. Drug interactions are common, and polypharmacy, defined by regular use of 5 or more medications, is present in 20–40% older adults on admission to the hospital. Additionally, potentially inappropriate prescribing of medications places the elderly at risk for adverse reactions. Unfortunately, nearly 35% of medication trials exclude older adult patients based on age alone. Therefore, the effect of aging on pharmacokinetics and pharmacodynamics of common drugs is often incompletely characterized and thus unpredictable [22].

General principles of acute pain treatment in older hospitalized patients utilize a multidisciplinary approach that combines pharmacologic and non-pharmacologic modalities with the goal of maximizing functional status for the patient and anticipating and managing treatment side effects [23]. Pain is an interaction between excitatory and inhibitory neurological pathways that integrate information from nociceptive, inflammatory, neuropathic, and emotional components; successful treatment strategies thus often require coordination of efforts directed at different components [8].

Although the mainstay of treatment for acute pain is pharmacotherapy, its effectiveness is greatly enhanced by patient education and multimodality interventions, such as physical therapy (PT), psychosocial support, and complementary and alternative treatments. The key to successful pain management is frequent assessment and treatment targeted to the type of pain. The World Health Organization (WHO) Analgesic Ladder was developed in 1986 and remains a widely used tool to address the management of cancer and non-cancer pain [24]. In step 1, WHO recommends the use of non-opioid analgesics with and without adjuvants for mild pain. In step 2, WHO recommends adding weaker opioids with or without adjuvants for moderate pain. In step 3, stronger opioids are added to the above drugs for severe pain. Commonly used adjuvants include topicals (lidocaine patch, capsaicin), acetaminophen, nonsteroidal anti-inflammatory drugs (NSAIDs), steroids, PT, heat/cold pack, massage, transcutaneous electrical nerve stimulation (TENS), etc. Neuropathic pain is surprisingly common in the hospital setting. Its prevalence is grossly underestimated, and as a result, it is undertreated. Table 2 provides resources for recommendations that have been suggested for specific types of pain.

Table 2 Resources for inpatient acute pain management

Class	Topic	Source of recommendations	Website or reference
General	Acute Pain Management	Australian and New Zealand College of Anaesthetists (2015)	Acute Pain Management: Scientific Evidence (2015). https://fpm.anzca.edu.au/documents/fpm-apmse4-final-20160426-v1-0.pdf
	Core Competencies in Pain Management	AAMC and all major pain professional societies	http://onlinelibrary.wiley.com/doi/10.1111/pme.12107/full *Pain Med.* 2013;14(7):971–81. https://doi.org/10.1111/pme.12107
Perioperative management	Specific procedures, e.g., TKR	PROSPECT	www.postoppain.org
	General Practice Guidelines	American Society of Anesthesiologists Task Force on Acute Pain Management	Practice-guidelines-for-acute-pain-management-in-the-perioperative-setting.pdf *Anesthesiology.* 2012;116(2):248–73. https://doi.org/10.1097/ALN.0b013e31823c1030
	Guidelines for Perioperative Management	Enhanced Recovery After Surgery (ERAS ®)	http://erassociety.org.loopiadns.com/guidelines/list-of-guidelines/
Quality/safety	Safe Opioid Use	The Joint Commission	Sentinel event alert issue 49: Safe use of opioids in hospitals, August 8, 2012. http://www.jointcommission.org/assets/1/18/SEA_49_opioids_8_2_12_final.pdf

Table 2 (continued)

Class	Topic	Source of recommendations	Website or reference
	Pain Assessment/ Management (Nursing)	Registered Nurses Association of Ontario	Assessment and Management of Pain, Third Edition (December, 2013) http://rnao.ca/sites/rnao-ca/files/AssessAndManagementOfPain2014.pdf
Medical	Guidelines for ICU	American College of Critical Care Medicine	Barr J, Fraser GL, Puntillo K, Ely EW, Gélinas C, Dasta JF, et al. Clinical practice guidelines for the management of pain, agitation, and delirium in adult patients in the intensive care unit. Crit Care Med. 2013;41(1):263–306. https://doi.org/10.1097/CCM.0b013e3182783b72.
	Opioid Overdose Prevention Toolkit (2016)	Substance Abuse and Mental Health Services Administration (SAMHSA)	https://store.samhsa.gov/product/Opioid-Overdose-Prevention-Toolkit-Updated-2016/SMA16-4742
	Pharmacologic management of neuropathic pain	National Institute for Health and Care Excellence	NICE Clinical Guideline 173 (Issued November 2013, updated February 2017). https://www.nice.org.uk/guidance/cg173/evidence/full-guideline-pdf-191621341
	Low back pain	Institute for Clinical Systems Improvement	Low Back Pain, Adult, Acute and Subacute (2012, undergoing revision) https://www.icsi.org/guidelines__more/catalog_guidelines_and_more/catalog_guidelines/catalog_musculoskeletal_guidelines/low_back_pain/
Instruments	APS-POQ-R (multiple languages)	American Pain Society	http://americanpainsociety.org/education/2010-revised-outcomes-questionnaire
	Visual Analogue Pain Scale (multiple languages)	British Pain Society	https://www.britishpainsociety.org/british-pain-society-publications/pain-scales-in-multiple-languages/
	Pain assessment tools for nonverbal older adults	City of Hope Pain & Palliative Care Resource Center	http://prc.coh.org/PAIN-NOA.htm
	Prescriber resources and assessment tools	Scope of Pain Opioid prescribing education	https://www.scopeofpain.com/tools-resources/

Management of Fracture or Surgery-Related Pain

The clinical scenario described earlier in this chapter highlights the challenges of managing pain in patients hospitalized with fractures. Effective pain control is an important aspect of the management of surgical patients. Preemptive pain management may reduce subsequent pain in the days to weeks following surgery. Greater pain control has the potential to allow for earlier hospital discharge and may improve the patient's ability to tolerate physical therapy. Postoperative pain may be undertreated in older patients, and opioid analgesics are often prescribed hesitantly in this population because of fear of adverse events. Another challenge to managing pain in this patient population is that a substantial proportion have cognitive impairment (from dementia, delirium, or both) and assessing pain requires aforementioned additional tools that may not be familiar to clinicians. Finally, effective pain prevention and treatment have both global and procedure-specific components; interventions that are effective in one circumstance may not be effective in others. Table 2 provides links and references that offer both general and specific guidelines.

Example: Hip Fractures Patients who experience greater pain are at higher risk for delirium, immobilization, prolonged hospitalization, and poorer health-related quality of life and report persistent pain 3–6 months after hip fracture [25]. A recent systematic review analyzed the best evidence on the effectiveness and safety of pharmacologic and non-pharmacologic techniques for managing pain in older adults after acute hip fracture [26]. In this analysis, moderate evidence suggests that nerve blockades are effective for relieving acute pain and reducing delirium, while low-level evidence suggests that preoperative traction does not reduce acute pain. Evidence was insufficient on the benefits and harms of most acute pain interventions [26], including spinal anesthesia, systemic analgesia, multimodal pain management, acupressure, relaxation therapy, TENS, and physical therapy regimens.

General Principles A recent high-quality review found that the best predictors of postoperative pain and analgesic consumption include preoperative pain, anxiety, age, and type of surgery [27]. Acute postoperative pain is best managed through a multimodal and preemptive analgesic approach [28]. For patients with prolonged surgery or with extensive incisions or who are on chronic opioids, neuraxial analgesia provided by spinal or epidural anesthesia with either morphine or fentanyl is recommended to decrease postoperative analgesic requirement. These techniques involve the introduction of local anesthetics and/or opiates into the distribution of certain spinal as well as peripheral nerves preoperatively. Regional techniques can block or reduce pain anywhere from several hours to several days, depending on the technique that is used. Peripheral nerve block has also been successfully used in trauma-related somatic pain such as hip fracture [26].

The American Society of Anesthesiologists (ASA) recently updated its practice guideline for acute pain management in the perioperative setting [29].

Its general recommendations call for appropriate institutional policies and procedures for providing perioperative pain management and patient education and the use of multimodal pain management therapy whenever possible. This approach includes preemptive analgesia, around-the-clock regimen of NSAIDs, COXIBs, or acetaminophen; regional blockade with local anesthetics; epidural and intrathecal opioids; and systemic opioid PCA, which is the preferred mode of postoperative pain control and leads to improved analgesic efficacy and patient satisfaction compared to nurse- or staff-administered opioids [28, 29]. The ASA's specific recommendations for special considerations for older patients are summarized in Table 3.

Perioperative Pain and Delirium: Walking the Tightrope

Postoperative pain is often overwhelming in its severity, and yet aggressive pain control may be hazardous and unnerving for the clinician. Avoiding oversedation and other drug-related side effects while maximizing comfort takes flexibility and vigilance. Certain basic tenets must be kept in mind:

- Postoperative pain is associated with an increased risk of delirium [30–32].
- Meperidine is the only opioid that has been clearly associated with delirium. Otherwise, there is no evidence to support one opioid over another [33].
- High-dose opioids may increase the risk of delirium, but the data are poor.
- Regional blocks may also reduce the risk of delirium [34].

The goal is to achieve balance – to relieve pain with opioids as needed while using creative strategies to avoid their overuse. We suggest the following strategy in surgical patients:

1. *Those who are performing the perioperative assessment should provide background information about the patient's comorbidities, – especially functional, affective and cognitive status – and talk directly with the anesthesiologist, whenever possible.*

Table 3 Recommendations regarding pain management in older persons from the American Society of Anesthesiologists Guidelines [29]

"Pain assessment and therapy should be integrated into the routine perioperative care of the older patients"
"Pain assessment tools appropriate to a patient's cognitive abilities should be used. Extensive and proactive evaluation and questioning may be necessary"
"Anesthesiologists should recognize that the older patients may respond differently than younger patients to pain and analgesic medications, often because of comorbidity"
"Vigilant dose titration is necessary to ensure adequate treatment while avoiding adverse effects such as somnolence in this vulnerable group, who are often taking many other medications (including alternative and complementary agents)"

If circumstances preclude it, document these needs clearly in the medical record. This will enable the anesthesiologist to choose medications and delivery methods that are safest and most effective [34, 35].
2. *Aim for adequate but not complete pain control.*
    A pain score of 1–3 is acceptable perioperatively. The patient must be able to get out of bed, participate in therapy, breathe deeply and effectively, sleep, and feel a sense of progress. Complete pain control is rarely achievable or necessary [34, 35].
3. *Prescribe the lowest dose of opioid required to achieve adequate analgesia.*
    (a) Use opioid-sparing adjuvants such as acetaminophen and NSAIDs [36], if not contraindicated by comorbidities or surgical procedure, and local treatments such as ice. Trials of individual drugs are enabling more specific therapeutic medication recommendations. Some examples: A recent large randomized, placebo-controlled trial of perioperative gabapentin in noncardiac surgery showed that it did not reduce the incidence of postoperative delirium or hospital length of stay, even though postoperative opioid dose was reduced significantly [37]. On the other hand, a recent large randomized, placebo-controlled trial of a non-opioid analgesic, dexmedetomidine, showed that low prophylactic dose significantly reduced incidence of delirium for elderly patients in the ICU after noncardiac surgery without significant side effects [38].
    (b) Prescribe standing small doses of opioids that the patient may refuse or that may be held if the patient is sedated. Do not prescribe postoperative opioids on an as-needed (prn) basis.
    (c) Consider patient-controlled analgesia (PCA), but only in those patients with the cognitive capacity to use it. A diagnosis of dementia is not a contraindication to PCA (nor is absence of dementia a guarantee that the patient will understand how to use this device). If there is any doubt, the patient should be asked to demonstrate where the button is, how to use it, and what it is for [11, 39].
4. *Reevaluate opioid needs frequently.*
    After several days, it may be possible to continue on standing acetaminophen with prn opioids before physical therapy and dressing changes.
5. *Reassess any new onset pain, especially in the back, pelvis, abdomen, or hips.*
    Ensure that pain in these sites is not due to constipation or urinary retention; in these cases, increasing the opioid dose will only exacerbate the underlying problem and, paradoxically, worsen the pain.

Acute Pain Management in Medical Inpatients

There is remarkably little literature on the management of acute pain in medical patients [40]. The challenges in older patients include liver and kidney dysfunction that leads to altered pharmacokinetics, altered pain perception, the need to individualize pain assessment tools, and the frequent superimposition of depression and altered cognition on painful states. Perhaps the greatest challenge is educating clinicians on the need to adjust the approach to pain management (especially opioid use) in this special population, with attention to the following general principles [23, 41]:

- Although there is wide interindividual variability in response to both the analgesic and adverse effects, no one opioid is superior to another.
- The routes of administration are PO, PR, IV, SQ, transdermal, or intraspinal. IM is discouraged, due to variable bioavailability; SQ is as effective as IV.
- Short-acting opioids are generally recommended when opioid therapy is being initiated for the first time or when the pain intensity is highly variable. Once stable, patients can be switched to a controlled-release or slow-release formulation.
- The initial opioid dose finding for acute pain is largely patient-driven, as determined by the balance of analgesia with side effects. The minimal starting dose is based on patient age and body weight, usually ranging from 0.05 to 0.1 mg/kg for IV morphine or from 0.0075 to 0.015 mg/kg for hydromorphone (lower limits usually apply to elderly patients). If no adequate pain relief is achieved within 15–30 min, a second or third dose can be given, and the effective analgesic dose will be the sum of the doses.
- The severity of the pain and the opioid formulation chosen determines the rate of titration. The dose of immediate-release formulation can be adjusted instantly, while long-acting opioids (Transdermal Fentanyl or methadone) can be adjusted daily or every 2 to 3 days. For mild-to-moderate pain, a dose increase of 25–50% is desired, while for severe and uncontrolled pain, a dose increase of 50–100% is appropriate.
- Opioid switching is a technique used to overcome inadequate pain control and dose-limiting toxic side effects, since there is a wide interindividual variability in response. The current guideline recommends calculating the equianalgesic amount and reducing the total dose by 25–50% to account for incomplete cross-tolerance.
- Most patients with constant pain require fixed-schedule dosing, along with as-needed rescue dosing for breakthrough pain, typically calculated at 10–20% of the total fixed dose.
- Patient-controlled analgesia (PCA), where the patient self-administers analgesics, offers patient convenience and enables rapid calculation of daily analgesia requirement.
- The key to safe use of PCA is close monitoring and adjustment with ready availability of naloxone. Every institution should set up its own monitoring parameters. Continuous infusion should be used with extreme caution in older patients, those who are obese, and those who have sleep apnea.

Neuropathic pain in medical inpatients usually results from damage to or dysfunction of a nerve, in contrast to activation of nociceptors in somatic and visceral pain. Neuropathic pain is common in patients with diabetes, shingles, herniated disks, multiple sclerosis, and AIDS. It is also commonly seen after surgery, radiation, or chemotherapy. Neuropathic pain may be resistant to standard opioid therapies or other nociceptive pain treatment strategies. Anticonvulsants and tricyclic antidepressants are mainstays of therapy. Complaints of continuous burning may respond best to antidepressants, whereas lancinating complaints may respond best to anticonvulsants. A recent review of published guidelines suggested first-line therapy for neuropathic pain includes TCAs, dual serotonin and norepinephrine inhibitors, gabapentin, pregabalin, and topical lidocaine, all of which are based on strong evidence from RCTs [42]. Opioids and tramadol are second-line therapy, and topical capsaicin, certain antidepressants and anticonvulsants, mexiletine, and NMDA receptor antagonists are third-line therapies. Chemotherapy-induced peripheral neuropathy is unique in that it responds poorly to TCAs and anticonvulsants. SNRIs such as duloxetine are the first-line therapy, followed by NSAIDs and opioids. In HIV neuropathy, antidepressants usually are ineffective, while topical capsaicin is modestly effective. These treatment modalities have been systematically reviewed [42].

When caring for aging medical inpatients, physicians should pay attention to traditional geriatric principles of medication management, which means starting low and titrating slowly [21–23]. It is reasonable to start opioids at 50–75% of the dose normally given to younger adults. It is imperative that the pain and pain medications, in particularly opioids, be monitored carefully in the elderly. In addition, non-pharmacologic treatments of pain, such as rehabilitation, physical therapy, adjuvant, and alternative and comprehensive therapy, should be emphasized to prevent functional decline in the hospital. Finally, treating acute pain in patients who are on chronic opioids remains challenging, and careful opioid initiation and titrating under expert guidance are required to avoid under- and overtreatment [43].

Acute Pain Management in the Nursing Home

The nursing home illustrates several challenges to the management of acute pain. Most skilled nursing facilities support a mix of residents: (1) those in long-term care and (2) those in subacute or short-term rehabilitation. Their pain needs are different, and staff must be prepared to respond appropriately.

Nursing home residents are assessed on a regular basis using a standardized tool, called the Minimum Data Set (MDS). The MDS 3.0, which has been in place since 2010, includes a pain interview that asks a resident if any pain has been present within the last 5 days, and if so, its frequency, whether it limits sleep or activity, and its severity (either verbal or numerical) [44]. Staff observations about a resident's pain, using a checklist of resident behaviors, are substituted if the resident cannot be interviewed. The MDS 3.0 also has questions about pain medications (scheduled and prn) and non-pharmacologic management of pain. The MDS data are used on site for resident care planning and quality improvement, and they are reported back to CMS.

The addition of pain interviews to the MDS 3.0 is an attempt to address concerns that pain in demented patients is not recognized or treated as aggressively as it is in those whose cognition is intact. There is nothing fundamentally different about pain management principles for those living in long-term care, once one takes comorbidities into account. In fact, that the resident lives on site and can be reassessed frequently should enable a more rapid and effective response to pain. It is all a matter of being alerted to changes in status and changing the plan of care accordingly.

Many residents admitted from the hospital for subacute rehabilitation will have acute pain: nonspecific trauma from falls, fragility fractures (hip, upper extremity, vertebra), postoperative discomfort, chest or pleuritic pain from pneumonia, and other causes. They will likely come with discharge instructions for pain management (or a list of the medications they were receiving), but the transfer to subacute rehabilitation necessitates a reassessment of the medication regimen:

- The facility's formulary may not include the medications the patient received in the hospital.
- The resident will be much more active and may suffer a temporary increase in pain intensity or frequency.
- The resident may have emotional responses to the illness or the transfer itself (e.g., fearing the less intensive monitoring outside of the acute setting or worrying about never going home) that may impair their coping strategies.
- Residents undergoing rehabilitation can expect to have frequent changes in their pain regimens as they are encouraged to do more and as they recover from their acute illness.
- At the time of discharge home, residents should have a supply of pain medication that is adequate to control pain for a week, in order to give them sufficient time to transition to their primary care provider or their surgeon for pain management.

Residents who develop acute pain in a long-term care facility should be quickly assessed and treated. Clinicians must decide if the resident must be transferred to an ED or can be treated locally. The development of acute pain has implications beyond the pain itself. It may signify a new change in the resident's status – a fracture, a new serious infection – that can affect the resident's future functional status and mortality. Nonetheless, it is essential to avoid reflexive transfer to the hospital if the pain can and should be managed locally. In addition, the following concerns must be addressed:

- The goals of care
  - Has there been a request to avoid hospitalization if at all possible, or is transfer to acute care expected if the patient has a serious illness?
  - How is the resident going to respond to an ED stay and subsequent hospitalization?
- The cause of the pain
  - If the resident has fallen, has there been a fracture? How is that to be definitively determined?
  - If the pain is chest or abdominal, can it be diagnosed safely and quickly?

- The treatment of the pain
  - If no surgical intervention is recommended (e.g. for repair of a hip fracture), can the pain be managed in the facility?
  - If the pain is due to an acute medical illness, can the illness itself be treated in the facility?
- The availability of palliative care and counseling services
  - If the treating team, (resident), and family feel that the resident is best off in the SNF, is there personnel trained to help the family cope with the decision to palliate rather than treat aggressively?

Quality Improvement in Acute Pain Management

Quality inpatient pain management is one of the core competencies for hospital-based practitioners [45]. Despite extensive research and quality improvement efforts in the last few decades, many barriers to high-quality inpatient pain management still exist. Moreover, interventions aimed at reducing these barriers have not been consistently shown to improve pain outcomes [40]. Systemic studies examining the quality of pain management in medical inpatients are scarce and areas of greatest uncertainty include:

- *How to treat acute pain quickly and effectively*
- Many feel that physicians and other providers should address acute pain episodes as medical emergencies, but how? A study from our own institution reveals frequent, prolonged severe pain episodes despite high rate of pain assessment, especially in chronic opioid users, suggesting an element of undertreatment [46]. On the other hand, acute pain teams and rapid response pain teams, led by either physicians or nurses, have not been shown to improve pain outcome [41, 47].
- *How to treat acute pain in the setting of chronic pain*
- These patients are likely to suffer increased frequency, severity, and duration of severe pain, with more marked functional consequences. This finding may be explained by the altered pain perceptions and maladaptive physiologic responses caused by the underlying chronic pain. Alternatively, chronic opioid users may have developed tolerance and subsequently require higher doses or more potent opiates, which is a practice that generates fear, uncertainty, and misconceptions among providers. Irrespective of mechanism, management of these patients' pain is especially difficult [43].
- *How to measure quality of treatment of acute pain*
- The Revised American Pain Society Patient Outcome Questionnaire (APS-POQ-R) is an example of a QI tool designed to measure the patient's impression of the quality of pain relief. It measures intensity, duration, emotional and functional impact, and side effects of medications. Despite being validated in several patient populations, the APS-POQ-R questionnaire has not yet been used extensively in inpatient settings as a quality improvement tool [48, 49]. Although the APS has recommended core quality indicators to measure the processes and out-

comes of pain management [48], direct measurements of these indicators might prove difficult; the APS-POQ-R questionnaire may be integrated into EHR and used as a surrogate marker of quality pain management.
- *How to design interventions to improve pain management*
- The design of a pain management intervention should aim to reduce overall pain scores at the system level, decrease pain-related medical errors, increase patient satisfaction, and reduce length of stay, cost, and inpatient mortality [50]. Most importantly, the process of pain management requires close interprofessional collaboration, active patient involvement, as well as an efficiently designed system of care. With the exception of patient education, which has been shown in small studies to improve outcomes (mostly through improvements in pain reporting and opioid prescribing), targeting individual components of pain management such as provider education, system-based pain assessment, algorithm or clinical pathway-based decision support systems, and dedicated pain management services has not been shown to improve clinical outcomes or quality of care consistently [50, 51]. Moreover, most of the pain management QI efforts have concentrated on the pain in the postoperative and orthopedic setting. In the orthopedic setting, several studies have shown that an interdisciplinary, multifaceted, protocol-driven pain management strategy reduces acute pain scores and health and hospitalization related cost in older hip fracture patients [52, 53]. In addition, untreated pain is being targeted as a medical error, either by chart auditing and feedback or real-time alert system through the EHR [54, 55]. These efforts have not been shown to reduce the overall pain score, however, despite an increased knowledge and prescription of pain medications. All these results suggest that any successful intervention would likely need to target all stakeholders in the process, while simultaneously addressing any systemic barriers commonly associated with institutional culture [56].

Summary and Outlook

Despite decades of clinical advances, research efforts, and public advocacy, achieving high-quality pain management remains difficult for the majority of patients, especially in acute institutional settings. This has been highlighted even more with the recent legal, ethical, and political debates about opioid abuse, misuse, and overdose-related mortality, as the United States is in the midst of a prescription opioid epidemic. Although the efforts to improve pain management are well intentioned, there are concerns that the pendulum has swung too far in the opposite direction [57, 58]. Clinicians managing acute pain are likely caught in the middle of needing to prioritize patient-perceived adequate pain control in the short term while balancing the potential long-term consequences of opioid use at discharge, as suggested in a 2015 survey of hospital physicians managing pain and opioid prescription [59].

Given the complexity and associated risks, as well as its direct impact on patient satisfaction, clinical providers must strive to achieve a certain level of competency for managing acute pain for institutionalized, elderly patients. In this regard, American Association of Medical Colleges (AAMC), along with all major professional societies on pain and pain management, recently established consensus-derived core competencies for pain management. They advocate for competency-based education at all levels, as well as for increased interprofessional collaboration and education in pain assessment and management [45]. These competencies fall within the following four essential domains:

- Multidimensional nature of pain
- Pain assessment and measurement
- Management of pain
- The context of pain management

While the guideline is not specific to the elderly population, its underlying principles align well with core geriatric principles of multifactorial assessment and treatment, avoidance of polypharmacy, goal settings, and transitions of care. Readers are also referred to a recent summary of evidences for pain treatment modalities in the elderly [23].

References

1. Gregory J, McGowan L. An examination of the prevalence of acute pain for hospitalized adult patients: a systemic review. J Clin Nurs. 2016;25:583–98.
2. Gianni W, Madaio RA, Di Cioccio L, et al. Prevalence of pain in elderly hospitalized patients. Arch Gerontol Geriatr. 2010;51:273–6.
3. Cascinu S, Giordani P, Agostinelli R, et al. Pain and its treatment in hospitalized patients with metastatic cancer. Support Care Cancer. 2003;11:587–92.
4. Whelan CT, Jin L, Meltzer D. Pain and satisfaction with pain control in hospitalized medical patients. Arch Intern Med. 2004;164:175–80.
5. Morris AC, Howie N. Pain in medical inpatients: an under-recognized problem? J R Coll Physicians Edinb. 2009;39:292–5.
6. Marks RM, Sachar EJ. Undertreatment of medical inpatients with narcotic analgesics. Ann Intern Med. 1973;78:173–81.
7. Cohen MZ, Easley MK, Ellis C, et al. Cancer pain management and the JCAHO's pain standards: an institutional challenge. J Pain Symptom Manag. 2003;25:519–27.
8. Woolf CJ. Pain: moving from symptom control toward mechanism-specific pharmacologic management. Ann Intern Med. 2004;140:441–51.
9. Clark D. 'Total pain', disciplinary power and the body in the work of Cicely Saunders, 1958–1967. Soc Sci Med. 1999;49:727–36.
10. Fortner BV, Demarco G, Irving G, et al. Description and predictors of direct and indirect costs of pain reported by cancer patients. J Pain Symptom Manag. 2003;25:9–18.
11. Mehta SS, Siegler EL, Henderson CR Jr, Reid MC. Acute pain management in hospitalized patients with cognitive impairment: a study of provider practices and treatment outcomes. Pain Med. 2010;11:1516–24.
12. Kelley AS, Siegler EL, Reid MC. Pitfalls and recommendations regarding the management of acute pain among hospitalized patients with dementia. Pain Med. 2008;9:581–6.
13. Orces CH. Emergency department visits for fall-related fractures among older adults in the USA: a retrospective cross-sectional analysis of the National Electronic Injury Surveillance System all injury program, 2001–2008. BMJ Open. 2013;3:e001722.

14. Platts-Mills TF, Esserman DA, Brown DL, et al. Older US emergency department patients are less likely to receive pain medication than younger patients: results from a national survey. Ann Emerg Med. 2012;60:199–206.
15. Hwang U, Richardson LD, Harris B, Morrison RS. The quality of emergency department pain care for elder adult patients. J Am Geriatr Soc. 2010;58:2122–8.
16. Cinar O, Ernst R, Fosnocht D, et al. Geriatric patients may not experience increased risk of oligoanalgesia in the emergency department. Ann Emerg Med. 2012;60:207–11.
17. Holland WC, Hunold KM, Mangipudi SA, et al. A prospective evaluation of shared-decision making regarding analgesics selection for older emergency department patients with acute musculoskeletal pain. Acad Emerg Med. 2016;23:306–14.
18. Hwang U, Platts-Mills TF. Acute pain management in older adults in the emergency department. Clin Geriatr Med. 2013;29:151–64.
19. Hogan TM, Howell MD, Cursio JF, et al. Improving pain relief in elder patients (I-PREP): an emergency department education and quality intervention. J Am Geriatr Soc. 2016;64:2566–71.
20. Kaye AD, Baluch A, Scott JT. Pain management in the elderly population: a review. Ochsner J. 2010;10:179–87.
21. Society of Hospital Medicine: Improving Pain Management for Hospitalized Patients Implementation Guide. Accessed on 8/12/17. http://www.hospitalmedicine.org/Web/Quality_Innovation/Implementation_Toolkits/Pain_Management/Web/Quality___Innovation/Implementation_Toolkit/Pain_Management_/Overview.aspx.
22. Ferrell BA. Pain management in elderly people. J Am Geriatr Soc. 1991;39:64–73.
23. Cornelius R, Herr KA, Gordon DB, Kretzer K. Acute pain management in older adults. J Gerontol Nurs. 2017;43:18–27.
24. Meldrum ML. A capsule history of pain management. JAMA. 2003;290:2470–5.
25. Herrick C, Steger-May K, Sinacore DR, et al. Persistent pain in frail older adults after hip fracture repair. J Am Geriatr Soc. 2004;52:2062–8.
26. Abou-Setta AM, Beaupre LA, Rashiq S, et al. Comparative effectiveness of pain management interventions for hip fracture: a systemic review. Ann Intern Med. 2011;155:234–45.
27. Wu CL, Raja SN. Treatment of acute postoperative pain. Lancet. 2011;377:2215–25.
28. Lovich-Sapola J, Smith CE, Brandt CP. Postoperative pain control. Surg Clin North Am. 2015;95:301–18.
29. American Society of Anesthesiologists. Practice guideline for acute pain management in the perioperative setting. Anesthesiology. 2012;116:248–73.
30. Lynch EP, Lazor MA, Gellis JE, et al. The impact of postoperative pain on the development of postoperative delirium. Anesth Analg. 1998;98:781–5.
31. Morrison RS, Magaziner J, Gilbert M, et al. Relationship between pain and opioid analgesics on the development of delirium following hip fracture. J Gerontol. 2003;58:76–81.
32. Vaurio LE, Sands LP, Wang Y, et al. Postoperative delirium: the importance of pain and pain management. Anesth Analg. 2006;102:1267–73.
33. Hong HK, Sands LP, Leung JM. The role of postoperative analgesia in delirium and cognitive decline in elderly patients: a systemic review. Anesth Analg. 2006;102:1255–66.
34. Rathier MO, Baker WL. A review of recent clinical trials and guidelines on the prevention and management of delirium in hospitalized older patients. Hosp Pract. 2011;39:96–106.
35. Marcantonio ER. Postoperative delirium. JAMA. 2012;308:73–81.
36. De Oliveira GS, Agarwal D, Benzon HT. Perioperative single dose ketorolac to prevent postoperative pain: a meta-analysis of randomized trials. Anesth Analg. 2012;114:424–33.
37. Leung JM, Sands LP, Chen N, Ames C, Berven S, Bozic K, et al. Perioperative gabapentin does not reduce postoperative delirium in older surgical patients: a randomized clinical trial. Anesthesiology. 2017;127(4):633–44.
38. Su X, Meng Z-T, Wu X-H, Cui F, Li H-L, Wang D-X, et al. Dexmedetomidine for prevention of delirium in elderly patients after non-cardiac surgery: a randomized, double-blind, placebo-controlled trial. Lancet. 2016;388:1893–902.
39. Licht E, Siegler EL, Reid MC. Can the cognitively impaired safely use patient-controlled analgesia? J Opioid Manag. 2009;5:307–12.

40. Helfand M, Freeman M. Assessment and management of acute pain in adult medical inpatients: a systemic review. Pain Med. 2009;10:1183–99.
41. Smith HS. Opioid metabolism. Mayo Clin Proc. 2009;84:613–24.
42. Dosenovic S, Jelicic Kadic A, Miljanovic M, Biocic K, Cavar M, Markovina N, et al. Interventions for neuropathic pain: an overview of systemic reviews. Anesth Analg. 2017;125:643–52.
43. Raub JN, Vettese TE. Acute pain management in hospitalized adult patients with opioid dependence: a narrative review and guide for clinicians. J Hosp Med. 2017;12:375–9.
44. Saliba D, Jones M, Streim J, et al. Overview of significant changes in the minimum data set for nursing homes version 3.0. JAMDA. 2012;13:595–601.
45. Fishman SM, Young HM, Arwood EL, et al. Core competencies for pain management: results of an interprofessional consensus summit. Pain Med. 2013;14:971–81.
46. Lin RJ, Reid MC, Chused AE, Evans AT. Quality assessment of acute inpatient pain management in an academic medical center. Am J Hosp Pallia Med. 2016;33:16–9.
47. Morrison RS, Meier DE, Fischberg D, et al. Improving the management of pain in hospitalized adults. Arch Intern Med. 2006;166:1033–9.
48. Gordon DB, Dahl JL, Miaskowski C, et al. American Pain Society recommendations for improving the quality of acute and cancer pain management. Arch Intern Med. 2005;165:1574–80.
49. Gordon DB, Polomano RC, Pellino TA, et al. Revised American Pain Society patient outcome questionnaire (APS-POQ-R) for quality improvement of pain management in hospitalized adults: preliminary psychometric evaluation. J Pain. 2010;11:1172–86.
50. Gordon DB, Dahl JL. Quality improvement challenges in pain management. Pain. 2004;107:1–4.
51. McNeill JA, Sherwood GD, Starck PL. The hidden error of mismanaged pain: a systems approach. J Pain Symptom Manag. 2004;28:47–58.
52. Brooks JM, Titler MG, Ardery G, Herr K. Effects of evidence-based acute pain management practices on in patient costs. Health Serv Res. 2009;44:245–63.
53. Titler MG, Herr K, Brooks JM, et al. Translating research into practice intervention improves management of acute pain in older hip fracture patient. Health Serv Res. 2009;44:264–87.
54. Hansson E, Fridlund B, Hallstrom I. Effects of a quality improvement program in acute care evaluated by patients, nurses, and physicians. Pain Manag Nurs. 2006;7:93–108.
55. Okon TR, Lutz PS, Liang H. Improved pain resolution in hospitalized patients through targeting of pain mismanagement as medical error. J Pain Symptom Manag. 2009;37:1039–49.
56. Lin RJ, Reid MC, Liu LL, Chused AE, Evans AT. The barriers to high-quality inpatient management: a qualitative study. Am J Hosp Pallia Med. 2016;32:594–9.
57. Beletsky L, Rich JD, Walley AY. Prevention of fatal opioid overdose. JAMA. 2012;308:1863–4.
58. Baker DW. History of the Joint Commission's pain standards. JAMA. 2017;317:1117–8.
59. Calcaterra SL, Drabkin AD, Leslie SE, Doyle R, Koester S, Frank JW, et al. The hospitalist perspective on opioid prescribing: a qualitative analysis. J Hosp Med. 2016;11:536–42.

Suggested Reading

Smith EM, Pang H, Cirrincione C, et al. Effect of duloxetine on pain, function, and quality of life among patients with chemotherapy-induced painful peripheral neuropathy: a randomized clinical trial. JAMA. 2013;309:1359–67.

Unique Physiologic Considerations

Nina M. Bemben and Mary Lynn McPherson

The aging process involves physiologic changes that impact both the disposition and effect of drugs in the body as well as the pathology of pain. As the population ages, an understanding of these principles is essential to recognizing patients in pain and treating their symptoms effectively and appropriately. In this chapter, age-related physiologic changes and their impact on drug pharmacokinetics and pharmacodynamics will be discussed.

Age-Related Changes in Physiology

Age-related physiologic changes lead to alterations in organ function that can impact the assessment and perception of pain, in addition to drug pharmacokinetics and pharmacodynamics. Changes in physiology occur as a normal part of aging but may also be accelerated by concomitant disease states. Safe and effective treatment of pain in older adults requires knowledge of these physiologic factors and their impact on drug therapy.

Changes in Pain Perception and Assessment

As people age, their perception of pain changes. Gibson and colleagues conducted a meta-analysis and found that as age increases, the pain threshold, or tolerance for pain, also increases for particular types of pain [1]. Specifically, the threshold for

---

N. M. Bemben
Kaiser Permanente, Oakland, CA, USA

M. L. McPherson (✉)
Department of Pharmacy Practice and Science, University of Maryland School of Pharmacy, Baltimore, MD, USA
e-mail: mmcphers@rx.umaryland.edu

somatosensory pain increases with age, while the threshold for pressure pain decreases [1]. Interestingly, the threshold for heat pain is not affected by age [1].

Symptoms of *neurologic* disease may appear as early as age 50 years, and the resultant neurologic dysfunction can impair both pain assessment and treatment [2]. As patients age, neurons are not regenerated and are instead replaced by glial cells [2, 3]. The majority of neuronal loss occurs within the neocortex and hippocampus, specifically the locus ceruleus and substantia nigra; these areas may influence pain perception [3]. Along with neuronal loss, the number of synapses, receptors, and intracellular enzymes all decrease, leading to changes in neurological function [2]. The function of the neurological system is also impacted by a 28% decrease in cerebral blood flow in elderly patients [3]. In addition to age-related neurological decline, the presence of Alzheimer's disease, normal-pressure hydrocephalus, malignancies, CNS infections, metabolic disorders, Parkinson's disease, and vascular disorders may all influence pain perception; these diseases increase in prevalence as patients age [2, 4].

Impact on Pharmacokinetics

Pharmacokinetics describes the processes of drug absorption, distribution, metabolism, and elimination in the body [5, 6]. Aging effects these pharmacokinetic processes, resulting in changes in the effects of drugs. Consideration of these changing pharmacokinetic parameters is essential for safe medication use in older adults.

Absorption
How aging affects drug absorption depends upon the route of drug administration. The transdermal route of administration is more impacted by aging than the oral, intramuscular and intravenous routes [7]. Less is known about the impact of aging on the sublingual route. Finally, among older patients, the rate of drug delivery, rather than the total dose, has a greater effect on the efficacy and toxicity of drugs [8, 9].

Transdermal
Age-related changes in skin can have an important effect on the absorption of drugs administered via the transdermal route, such as fentanyl. As patients age, significantly less transdermal fentanyl is absorbed [5]. A study using human skin samples found that in patients over age 60 years, the absorption rate, area under the curve (AUC), lag time, and total amount of fentanyl absorbed from a transdermal patch decreased compared to younger patients [5]. Additionally, elderly and cachectic patients are at an increased risk of respiratory depression with transdermal fentanyl due to changes in pharmacokinetics [10].

Sublingual
The amount of saliva influences the absorption of drugs administered sublingually. The age-related decrease in saliva production can impact the absorption of

sublingual tablets or matrix-embedded drugs, such as buprenorphine [3]. In addition to age-related decreases in saliva production, polypharmacy is common in elderly patients and may result in dry mouth [11]. Polypharmacy itself may be more predictive of dry mouth than particular drugs; however some drugs are known to exacerbate dry mouth symptoms [11]. Examples of drugs commonly associated with dry mouth include diuretics, antihistamines, sympathomimetics, skeletal muscle relaxants, benzodiazepines, opioids, H2 receptor antagonists, cytotoxic drugs, retinoids, antiretrovirals, and cytokines [11].

Oral
The absorption of drugs administered orally generally occurs in the stomach or proximal intestine and is less impacted by age-related physiological changes than the transdermal or sublingual routes of administration [6, 7]. Additionally, small bowel absorption is not significantly affected by aging and is not a factor in drug efficacy [3].

Intramuscular
While intramuscular absorption is not as significantly impacted by aging as the transdermal route, elderly patients do generally have less muscle mass than younger patients.

Intravenous
No absorption is required for drugs administered via the intravenous route; hence the aging process does not affect this route of administration.

Distribution
The aging process leads to important physiological changes in body composition that affect the disposition of drugs in the body.

Lipophilic Drugs
As people age, there is an increase in body fat along with a decrease in muscle mass [7]. This results in an increased volume of distribution and elimination half-life (due to extensive tissue distribution) for lipophilic drugs such as fentanyl and methadone (see Table 1 for a description of opioid and metabolite half-lives) [3, 5, 12, 13].

Hydrophilic Drugs
Due to decreased muscle mass and total body water, hydrophilic drugs such as morphine and hydromorphone have a smaller volume of distribution, leading to increased serum concentrations compared to those seen in younger patients who receive the same dose [2, 3, 5, 13]. This smaller volume of distribution and resultant higher serum concentration for hydrophilic drugs may result in drug efficacy at lower doses than those typically used in younger patients. For the same reason, older patients may experience adverse effects with lower doses than those known to cause adverse effects in younger patients [2, 3].

Table 1 Opioid and metabolite half-lives [13]

Drug/metabolite	Plasma half-life (hours)
Short half-life opioids	
Morphine	2–3.5
Morphine-6 glucuronide	2
Hydromorphone	2–3
Oxycodone	2–3
Fentanyl	3–4
Codeine	3
Meperidine	3–4
Nalbuphine	5
Butorphanol	2.5–3.5
Buprenorphine	3–5
Long half-life opioids	
Methadone	24–150
Levorphanol	12–16
Normeperidine	14–21

Protein-Bound Drugs

An age-related decrease in the production of plasma proteins which bind drugs leads to increases in the free fraction (active component) of drugs that are extensively protein bound, such as NSAIDs, morphine, and antiepileptic drugs (AEDs) [2, 3]. As age increases, both the quantity and quality of albumin produced by the liver decreases, resulting in less albumin binding of drugs and more drug being free to exert its activity [2]. Thus, in an elderly patient with decreased albumin levels, the same dose of a highly albumin-bound drug, such as morphine, will have greater activity (both therapeutic and toxic) due to the higher free fraction of drug in the serum. Phenytoin is also highly bound to albumin, and patients with hypoalbuminemia will have falsely low total phenytoin levels when therapeutic drug monitoring is performed, potentially leading practitioners to falsely interpret those levels as therapeutic when in fact they are toxic. In contrast to the total phenytoin level, the free fraction of phenytoin (i.e., that fraction of drug not bound to albumin) will indeed be above the therapeutic range indicating potential toxicity. Hepatic albumin production may be further decreased in older adults with comorbidities such as malnutrition [2].

Metabolism

Elderly patients are generally more sensitive to both the therapeutic and toxic effects of drugs. This is due in part to age-related reduced metabolism. Although the liver metabolizes most drugs, elderly patients experience a striking 30–40% decline in hepatic function [2, 3, 14]. For example, after the age of 50 years, liver mass decreases by 1% per year so that patients over age 65 years have a 33% decrease in portal blood flow compared to younger patients [2, 3, 7, 15]. As hepatic function declines with age, phase 2 reactions (acetylation, glucuronidation, sulfation, glycine conjugation) decrease to a greater extent than phase 1 reactions (oxidation, hydrolysis, reduction) [2].

Specific age-related changes in metabolism may impact the activity of a variety of drugs used for analgesia. For example, an age-related decrease in demethylation can impair the metabolism of benzodiazepines, particularly those with a long duration of action such as clonazepam, diazepam, and chlordiazepoxide (see Table 2) [2, 16]. Glutathione conjugation is also decreased in the elderly, which can lead to a decrease in the inactivation of the toxic metabolite of acetaminophen, N-acetyl-p-benzoquinone imine (NAPQI), and thus an increased sensitivity to acetaminophen-induced hepatic toxicity [2]. Decreased glucuronidation activity can also increase the toxicity of morphine [2].

First-pass hepatic metabolism also decreases with age due to decreased hepatic portal and arterial blood flow [2, 3, 12]. As a result, adverse effects appear at lower doses of drugs such as lidocaine, which typically undergo extensive first-pass metabolism [2]. Some opioids, such as buprenorphine and hydromorphone, also undergo extensive first-pass metabolism, and thus adverse effects may be expected at lower doses in older patients, as they are exposed to more active drug [13]. In the case of hydromorphone, 62% of the drug is metabolized on first pass; therefore, among elderly patients with reduced first-pass metabolism, higher serum drug concentrations can be expected from the same dose when compared to younger patients in whom a greater fraction of drug is removed via first-pass metabolism [13].

Liver disease can further decrease hepatic metabolism [2]. Unlike renal function, there are no universal clinical tests of hepatic function; in fact, liver transaminases may be within the normal range in patients with liver disease or cirrhosis [2, 12]. While the Child-Pugh score reliably assesses hepatic function and is recommended by the Food and Drug Administration (FDA) for use in clinical trials, liver impairment as described by the Child-Pugh score is not always directly correlated with an impact on drug pharmacokinetics [15]. Rather than relying solely on laboratory data or the Child-Pugh score to assess liver function, clinicians should consider risk factors for hepatic impairment (such as alcohol abuse, chronic hepatitis B or C, biliary tract obstruction, biliary cirrhosis, hemochromatosis, and morbid obesity) when selecting drug therapy [15].

Table 2 Benzodiazepine duration of action [32]

Benzodiazepines with short and intermediate durations of action	Alprazolam
	Bromazepam
	Clonazepam
	Lorazepam
	Oxazepam
	Temazepam
Benzodiazepines with long duration of action	Clorazepate
	Chlordiazepoxide
	Diazepam
	Flurazepam

Excretion

In addition to an age-related decrease in drug metabolism, an age-related decrease in excretion due to declining renal function also predisposes elderly patients to drug adverse effects. Renal function decreases with increasing age at a rate of 1% per year after age 40, which impacts the clearance of many drugs and/or their metabolites [2, 3, 7, 14]. This decline is equivalent to a 1 mL/min decrease in creatinine clearance per year [2, 3]. The decline in renal function may be attributed to decreased renal blood flow; decreased kidney mass; and decrease in the number, length, and thickness of renal tubules [2]. In addition, free water absorption decreases after age 50 years, at a rate of 5% per 10 years [2]. Older adults produce less creatinine due to decreased muscle mass; thus measuring the serum creatinine does not accurately represent renal function in older adults, as decreased renal function can coexist with apparently normal serum creatinine levels [12]. However, estimates of renal function such as the glomerular filtration rate can account for age-related decreases in serum creatinine and give an accurate assessment of renal function in elderly patients. Age-related decline in renal function is accelerated in the presence of comorbidities such as hypertension, heart failure, and atherosclerosis [2].

Impact on Pharmacodynamics

Pharmacodynamics describe the relation between drug concentration at the site of action and the magnitude of the clinical effect [9]. Pharmacodynamic effects of drugs are dependent on drug dose and also on patient-specific factors such as concomitant disease states and medications which can raise or lower the threshold for achieving a drug effect. Elderly patients are more likely than younger patients to have multiple comorbidities and concomitant medications [17].

Changes in Drug Efficacy

Opioids are commonly used to treat pain, and they exert their effects by binding and activating opioid receptors. All opioid receptors belong to the G protein-coupled seven transmembrane receptor superfamily (GPCR) [18]. When an opioid agonist binds to an opioid receptor, a conformational change is induced, which leads to G-protein coupling and activation [18]. However, in elderly patients, an age-related decrease in the coupling of G-proteins may explain delayed opioid efficacy [2, 18]. In addition, adenylate cyclase is a secondary mediator of opioid agonist activity which has reduced activity in elderly patients [2, 18]. While delayed efficacy results in increased time to therapeutic effect, it does not necessarily mean reduced sensitivity to opioids and other centrally active agents. In fact, the physiological changes discussed above all contribute to an increased sensitivity to central nervous system (CNS) active drugs such as benzodiazepines and opioids among aging patients [2, 3, 12, 14, 16].

In addition to delayed opioid efficacy and increased sensitivity, elderly patients have also been shown to develop less tolerance to opioids than do younger patients [8, 18]. A retrospective chart review conducted in patients treated for chronic nonmalignant pain found patients aged 50 years or younger increased their dose of oral opioids at a rate more than double that of patients aged 60 years or older [19]. These differences in opioid dosing were not explained by pharmacokinetic parameters alone and were instead attributed to age-related changes in the development of opioid tolerance [19]. Animal studies have found that the increased cellular and molecular neuroplasticity seen in younger groups of patients contributes to a more rapid development of tolerance than that seen in older groups of patients [8]. Additionally, the expression and distribution of endogenous opioids, which serve to modulate pain, are age-related and may also be decreased in the elderly [8, 18].

Changes in Drug Adverse Effects

An age-related decrease in gastrointestinal peristalsis predisposes elderly patients to constipation. Opioids will cause constipation regardless of patient age and should be used with prophylactic bowel regimens in all patients; however elderly patients may require even more vigilance against constipation. Other medications commonly used for pain, such as the TCAs, are more likely to cause constipation in older adults due to their anticholinergic adverse effect profile. In addition to the age-related decrease in gastrointestinal peristalsis, elderly patients also experience a decline in the thirst reflex, predisposing them to dehydration, which can also exacerbate constipation [20].

Decreased response of baroreceptors commonly leads to orthostatic hypotension in elderly patients and can lead to falls [3]. Morphine may exacerbate orthostatic hypotension by decreasing sympathetic nervous system tone and causing histamine release, a common adverse effect [13]. Drugs commonly used to treat pain, such as tricyclic antidepressants (TCAs) and anticonvulsants, may also increase the risk of falls in elderly patients [2, 16]. The American Geriatrics Society recommends these medications be avoided in elderly patients with a history of falls or fractures unless safer alternatives are not available [16].

As patients age, the total body water decreases, predisposing elderly patients, particularly women, to hyponatremia [20]. In fact, by age 75–80 years, the total body water content is decreased by 50% in comparison to younger patients [20]. Carbamazepine, serotonin norepinephrine reuptake inhibitors (SNRIs), opioids, and TCAs are used commonly in pain management but may also cause or exacerbate syndrome of inappropriate antidiuretic hormone (SIADH) or hyponatremia [16, 20]. If these medications are used in the elderly, serum sodium levels must be monitored closely, particularly upon initiation and dosage increases [16].

Impact of Concomitant Disease States

Patients with cardiovascular disease, cerebrovascular disease, respiratory disease, sleep apnea, lung cancer, or patients who smoke ≥2 packs/day are more susceptible to opioid-induced respiratory depression compared to patients without these comorbidities [15]. Some data suggests that elderly patients, with or without the above comorbidities, are more sensitive than younger patients to the adverse effects of opioids, particularly respiratory depression [15]. Thus, in elderly patients and those with the comorbidities discussed above, a drug level which would not typically cause opioid-induced respiratory depression in a younger patient without comorbidities could in fact lead to respiratory depression. In addition to opioid-induced respiratory depression, patients with the above comorbidities are also at an increased risk of opioid-induced bradycardia and hypotension [15]. Cardiovascular disease, particularly heart failure, also increases risk of heart failure exacerbation with NSAID therapy [16].

Patients with comorbid cerebrovascular disease, dementia, brain injury, or psychiatric illness are at increased risk of CNS adverse effects with opioid therapy, including euphoria, dysphoria, cognitive impairment, delirium, hallucinations, and sedation [15]. The CNS adverse effects of opioids are particularly worrisome in elderly patients, and may be affected by the route of administration and onset of action of opioids (those agents with a faster onset of action being more likely to cause adverse CNS affects) [15]. Comorbid dementia or cognitive impairment also increases the risk of adverse CNS effects with drugs such as anticholinergics and benzodiazepines [16].

Due to age-related changes in physiology and the potential for pharmacodynamic changes to result in adverse effects, the American Geriatrics Society has developed a list of potentially inappropriate medications for use in elderly patients, known as the Beers list [16]. Many drugs used frequently in pain management appear on this list, and their use should be avoided in elderly patients (see recommendations for therapy, below).

Drug Interactions

The increase in comorbid conditions that occurs with aging increases the likelihood of polypharmacy, which can lead to drug-drug interactions [17]. Drug-drug interactions may be pharmacokinetic or pharmacodynamic in nature, and they may enhance or blunt the efficacy or toxicity of medications used to treat pain [14, 15]. Elderly patients are exposed to drug-drug interactions at a rate of 25–45% [21]. An appreciation of when drug-drug interactions are likely to occur and how they can be appropriately managed or avoided can help ensure patients achieve maximum benefit with minimal risk from their pain management regimen.

Pharmacokinetic Drug Interactions

Pharmacokinetic drug-drug interactions result when one drug interferes with the absorption, distribution, metabolism, or elimination of another drug. Most commonly, pharmacokinetic drug interactions are metabolic in nature, with one drug impacting another's metabolism via induction, inhibition, or competition for metabolism [6]. Selected major pharmacokinetic interactions for drugs commonly used in pain management are shown in Table 3.

Table 3 Selected major pharmacokinetic interactions for analgesics [22]

Analgesic	Interacting drug	Interaction effect and proposed mechanism	Clinical management
Amitriptyline	Fluconazole	Increased risk of amitriptyline toxicity due to inhibition of CYP-mediated amitriptyline metabolism	Use caution if both drugs are used concomitantly
	Fluoxetine	Increased risk of amitriptyline toxicity due to decreased amitriptyline metabolism	Concomitant use not recommended
	Sertraline	Increased serum levels of amitriptyline due to inhibition of amitriptyline metabolism	Use caution if both drugs are used concomitantly
Senna	Droperidol	Increased risk of QT prolongation and resulting torsades de pointes and cardiac arrest due electrolyte abnormalities. Prolonged or excessive use of senna may result in loss of potassium and magnesium	Use extreme caution with droperidol in patients taking concomitant senna
Fentanyl	Clarithromycin	Increased fentanyl-induced CNS and respiratory depression due to inhibition of CYP3A4-mediated fentanyl metabolism	Monitor patients for fentanyl toxicity and reduce fentanyl dose
	Diltiazem	Severe hypotension and increased risk of fentanyl-induced respiratory depression due to inhibition of CYP3A4-mediated fentanyl metabolism	Monitor blood pressure and reduce fentanyl dose if necessary
	Erythromycin	Increased fentanyl-induced CNS and respiratory depression due to inhibition of CYP3A4-mediated fentanyl metabolism	Monitor patients and reduce fentanyl dose
	Fluconazole	Increased fentanyl-induced CNS and respiratory depression due to inhibition of CYP3A4-mediated fentanyl metabolism	Monitor patients and reduce fentanyl dose
	Ketoconazole	Increased fentanyl-induced CNS and respiratory depression due to inhibition of CYP3A4-mediated fentanyl metabolism	Monitor patients and reduce fentanyl dose
Morphine	Cimetidine	Increased morphine toxicity possibly due to reduced morphine metabolism	Use cimetidine cautiously in patients taking morphine. Initiate morphine at lower doses
Tramadol	Carbamazepine	Decreased efficacy of tramadol due to carbamazepine induction of tramadol metabolism	Concurrent use of tramadol and carbamazepine not recommended

(continued)

Table 3 (continued)

Analgesic	Interacting drug	Interaction effect and proposed mechanism	Clinical management
Trazodone	Amiodarone	Increased risk of QT-interval prolongation and torsades de pointes due amiodarone inhibition of CYP3A4-mediated metabolism of trazodone. Amiodarone is also metabolized by CYP3A4 and competes with trazodone for metabolism	If trazodone and amiodarone are used concomitantly, use caution and monitor for signs of cardiotoxicity
	Fluoxetine	Increased risk of trazodone toxicity and serotonin syndrome due to reduced clearance of trazodone	Consider reduction in trazodone dose and monitor for toxicity

Reproduced by permission of Oxford University Press, USA

An example of a drug-drug interaction that interferes with the process of absorption occurs between mineral oil enemas and docusate, both of which could be used to manage opioid-induced constipation [22]. When used together, mineral oil enemas and docusate can result in increased mineral oil absorption resulting in gastrointestinal inflammation [22]. Due to this pharmacokinetic drug-drug interaction, the concurrent administration of mineral oil and docusate should be avoided [22]. In addition, because anticholinergic drugs such as TCAs and opioids delay gastric emptying, they can slow the onset of action of other concomitant medications [22]. Absorption of some drugs, such as gabapentin, requires an acidic environment [22]. Thus, medications that reduce gastric acidity, such as proton pump inhibitors (PPIs) and histamine-2-receptor antagonists, can interfere with the absorption of gabapentin [22].

Concomitant use of gabapentin and aluminum antacids can result in a drug-drug interaction due to changes in the distribution of gabapentin [22]. Aluminum binds gabapentin, resulting in decreased gabapentin efficacy due to decreased free gabapentin [22]. Due to this interaction, patients taking gabapentin should be advised to avoid using antacids [22].

Most opioids are metabolized by CYP2D6 and CYP3A4 [5, 15]. Over 50% of all drugs are metabolized by CYP3A4 leading to an increased likelihood of CYP-mediated drug-drug interactions as the number of medications increases [5, 15]. Codeine, hydrocodone, oxycodone, and methadone are all metabolized by CYP2D6; thus increased drug levels may be seen when used concomitantly with a CYP2D6 inhibitor such as the NSAID celecoxib [13, 15]. Methadone, fentanyl, and buprenorphine are primarily metabolized by CYP3A4, and concomitant use with CYP3A4 inhibitors or inducers such as ketoconazole and carbamazepine may lead to increased or decreased opioid levels, respectively [13, 15]. Levorphanol is an opioid agonist at the μ, κ, and δ opioid receptors and an antagonist at the NMDA receptor which has been proposed to have clinically important drug-drug interactions with NSAIDs, valproic acid, lorazepam, and rifampin [13]. When used in combination with monoamine oxidase inhibitors (MAOIs), meperidine can cause severe respiratory depression, hyperpyrexia, CNS excitation, delirium, and seizures [13]. For patients in whom pharmacokinetic drug-drug interactions present a challenge, selecting opioids that are metabolized predominantly by glucuronidation, rather than by CYP enzymes, can avoid many potentially problematic drug-drug interactions [15]. Morphine, hydromorphone, oxymorphone, and tapentadol all undergo glucuronidation and are not metabolized by the CYP enzyme system [15]. Tapentadol has been shown to be a weak inhibitor of CYP2D6, but this inhibition is not clinically significant [15].

In addition to metabolism, drug elimination may also be affected by concomitant drug therapy. In pain management, drug toxicity due to decreased elimination is most likely to occur due to age-related declines in renal function and resultant drug accumulation rather than pharmacokinetic drug-drug interactions [22]. However, one example of a pharmacokinetic drug interaction due to changes in elimination is the interaction of probenecid and methotrexate [22]. Probenecid impacts the renal secretion of drugs such as methotrexate and can cause methotrexate toxicity by decreasing its elimination [22].

Pharmacodynamic Drug Interactions

Pharmacodynamic drug-drug interactions are those related to additive, synergistic, or antagonistic drug effects. When more than one drug acting on the same biochemical pathway is used concomitantly, pharmacodynamic drug-drug interactions can occur. For example, in addition to activity at the μ opioid receptor, methadone also inhibits the reuptake of norepinephrine and serotonin in the central nervous system (CNS) and thus acts on the same biochemical pathway as serotonin-norepinephrine reuptake inhibitors (SNRIs) and tricyclic antidepressants (TCAs), both classes of medications commonly used in pain management [15]. Using methadone in combination with SNRIs or TCAs could lead to additive inhibition of serotonin reuptake resulting in excess serotonin availability in the CNS and the potential for serotonin syndrome. Serotonin syndrome symptoms can range from mild to life-threatening, including tremor, altered mental status, hyperthermia, and muscular hypertonicity [23]. Another example of pharmacodynamic interactions is the additive CNS depressive effects seen when opioids are used in combination with other CNS-active agents such as antidepressants, sedatives, and phenothiazines [15].

In addition to opioids, elderly patients may also be prescribed other medications commonly used for pain such as tricyclic antidepressants (TCAs) and skeletal muscle relaxants (i.e., carisoprodol, cyclobenzaprine, metaxalone, methocarbamol) which can exacerbate constipation and dry mouth in older adults due to their anticholinergic adverse effects [3, 11, 16]. Anticholinergic adverse effects include constipation, urinary retention, blurred vision, dry mouth, and cognitive impairment [24].

The use of nonsteroidal anti-inflammatory drugs (NSAIDs), which further decrease renin production in addition to the age-related decline, may exacerbate hypokalemia in elderly patients [3]. Hypokalemia can also increase the risk of

QT-interval prolongation and torsades de pointes, and this risk is further increased when QT-interval prolonging drugs such as methadone are used in elderly patients [13]. Thus, a pharmacodynamic drug-drug interaction can result when NSAIDs and methadone are used concomitantly, whereby the increased risk of hypokalemia with NSAIDs predisposes patients to the risk of QT-interval prolongation and torsades de pointes with methadone.

Recommendations for Therapy

Special considerations in drug therapy selection are needed for older adults, due to age-related changes in physiology, increased prevalence of concomitant disease states, and increased risk of drug-drug interactions. Older adults are more sensitive to the adverse effects of some medications commonly used to treat pain, such as NSAIDs and opioids. Avoidance of high-risk medications and drug-drug interactions can help reduce the risk of adverse effects while still providing appropriate pain management.

General Therapy Recommendations

Established criteria, such as the Beers Criteria developed by the American Geriatrics Society, identify drugs that are potentially inappropriate for use in older adults due to their adverse effect profile [16]. Those drugs which may be used in pain management and have been identified as potentially inappropriate for use in older adults include tertiary TCAs, benzodiazepines, meperidine, NSAIDs, pentazocine, and skeletal muscle relaxants (see Table 4) [16].

The tertiary TCAs include amitriptyline, clomipramine, imipramine, doxepin (in doses >6 mg/day), and trimipramine [16]. These drugs are considered potentially inappropriate for use in older adults due to their association with arrhythmias, syncope, falls, constipation, dry mouth, reduced clearance, and overdose potential [12, 16]. Secondary amine tricyclic antidepressants include desipramine, nortriptyline, and protriptyline, and they may be used in place of the tertiary amine TCAs in elderly patients and have been proposed to have a favorable adverse effect profile. However, a recent prospective study found nortriptyline, a secondary amine TCA, to be similarly tolerated by patients when compared to amitriptyline in patients with neuropathic pain [24].

Meperidine should also be avoided in older adults due to its potential for CNS adverse effects and neurotoxicity [12, 14, 16]. In addition, the doses of meperidine commonly used for oral analgesia are likely ineffective, and safer analgesic options exist [16]. Pentazocine, like meperidine, is another opioid that is not recommended for use in older adults due to the high prevalence of CNS adverse effects (confusion and hallucinations) and the availability of safer alternatives [16]. The American Geriatrics Society also recommends that skeletal muscle relaxants, such as carisoprodol, cyclobenzaprine, and methocarbamol, be avoided in elderly patients due to

Table 4 Medications commonly used in pain management identified as potentially inappropriate for older adults by Beers list [16]

Medication class	Safety concern

Tertiary TCAs
  Amitriptyline
  Clomipramine
  Doxepin >6 mg/day
  Imipramine
  Trimipramine
	Anticholinergic effects
	Sedation
	Orthostatic hypotension

Benzodiazepines	Cognitive impairment Delirium Increased fall risk
Meperidine	Potentially neurotoxic

Non-COX-selective NSAIDs
  Aspirin >325 mg/day
  Diclofenac
  Diflunisal
  Etodolac
  Fenoprofen
  Ibuprofen
  Ketoprofen
  Meclofenamate
  Mefenamic acid
  Meloxicam
  Nabumetone
  Naproxen
  Oxaprozin
  Piroxicam
  Sulindac
  Tolmetin
Indomethacin
Ketorolac
	Increased risk of GI bleeding in patients >75 years old or those taking corticosteroids, anticoagulants, or antiplatelets

Pentazocine	Confusion and hallucinations

Skeletal muscle relaxants
  Carisoprodol
  Chlorzoxazone
  Cyclobenzaprine
  Metaxalone
  Methocarbamol
  Orphenadrine
	Anticholinergic effects
	Sedation
	Increased risk of fracture
	Questionable efficacy at tolerable doses

their high prevalence of anticholinergic adverse effects (confusion, dry mouth, constipation) and questionable efficacy at tolerable doses [16]. For many years, propoxyphene was commonly used in older adults as an analgesic, and its use persisted even after it was identified as an inappropriate medication for elderly patients. However in 2010 propoxyphene was removed from the US market due to concerns regarding CNS adverse effects, cardiotoxicity, and potential for renal or hepatic toxicity [12, 14, 25].

All NSAIDs carry identical boxed warnings related to cardiovascular and gastrointestinal risk, regardless of patient age [26]. NSAIDs have been associated with an increased risk of thrombotic events such as myocardial infarction and stroke, and this risk may be further elevated in patients with existing cardiac disease or risk factors for cardiac disease [26]. Additionally, chronic use of non-COX-selective NSAIDs (i.e., aspirin >325 mg/day, diclofenac, diflunisal, etodolac, fenoprofen, ibuprofen, ketoprofen, meclofenamate, mefenamic acid, meloxicam, nabumetone, naproxen, oxaprozin, piroxicam, sulindac, tolmetin) in older adults is not recommended due to the increased risk of gastrointestinal bleeding and peptic ulcer disease in patients at high risk for these adverse effects [16]. High-risk patients include those over age 75 years and patients treated with corticosteroids, anticoagulants, or antiplatelets [16]. If other agents are ineffective and NSAIDs must be used in older adults, concomitant use with a proton pump inhibitor (PPI) or misoprostol is recommended to decrease the risk of gastrointestinal bleeding [16]. While using NSAIDs with a PPI or misoprostol decreases the risk of gastrointestinal toxicity, this risk cannot be eliminated [16]. Topical NSAIDs may be a safer option due to lower serum concentrations achieved when compared to systemic NSAIDs, although they still carry the same boxed warning regarding cardiovascular and gastrointestinal risks [28]. Of all the NSAID agents, indomethacin is associated with the highest risk of gastrointestinal bleeding and should be avoided specifically in elderly patients considered to be high risk [12, 16].

In addition to the risk of adverse cardiovascular and gastrointestinal effects, NSAIDs with a long duration of action, such as naproxen, oxaprozin, and piroxicam, should be avoided in elderly patients due to the risk of renal failure, hypertension, fluid retention, and heart failure [12, 16]. Due to the increased risk of kidney injury, NSAIDs should be avoided in patients with stage IV or V chronic kidney disease [16]. Elderly patients are also predisposed to hypokalemia due to age-related changes in renin production, which may be exacerbated by NSAIDs [3].

In older adult patients with concomitant respiratory or cardiovascular disease, methadone is more likely to cause QT-interval prolongation and may not be preferred for these patients [15]. Codeine has been associated with severe hypotension and respiratory depression and is also less suitable for patients with preexisting respiratory or cardiovascular disease [15]. Morphine may be an alternative to methadone and codeine in this case but should be used cautiously as the potential for respiratory depression still exists [15]. For patients requiring a less powerful opioid, tramadol is an alternative to codeine and NSAIDs, both of which should be avoided in these patients [15].

It is important to consider the duration of activity for a particular drug when designing a therapeutic regimen. For example, the analgesic effect of methadone is shorter in duration than respiratory depression, which could lead to potentially dangerous adverse effects if dosed too frequently or titrated too rapidly [14].

Elderly patients may be more likely than younger patients to have difficulty swallowing and taking drugs administered orally; parenteral, chewable, or oral disintegrating formulations would be desirable in these patients. Morphine, hydromorphone, and oxycodone are all available in rectal formulations, while fentanyl, hydromorphone, morphine, oxymorphone, and buprenorphine are all available as injectables [15]. Both fentanyl and buprenorphine are available as transdermal patches [10, 27]. Transmucosal fentanyl is available as both a buccal tablet and buccal soluble film; however these agents are only approved for use in breakthrough cancer pain in opioid-tolerant patients [29–32]. The intrathecal or epidural route can be used for fentanyl, morphine, and hydromorphone [15].

Benzodiazepines should be used cautiously in older adults due to their associated risks of cognitive impairment, delirium, and falls; however they may be appropriate in specific situations such as periprocedural anesthesia and end-of-life care [16]. The use of long-acting benzodiazepines in elderly patients may lead to sedation, cognitive impairment, and falls (see Table 2) [12]. Thus, if benzodiazepines must be used in older adults, those with a shorter duration of action are preferred.

Patients with Renal Impairment

Due to the age-associated decline in renal function, caution must be used when initiating therapy with drugs that are primarily renally excreted, such as gabapentin [2]. In addition, drugs with active metabolites that are primarily renally excreted, such as morphine, codeine, oxycodone, tramadol, and meperidine, should be used cautiously as these active metabolites may accumulate and lead to toxicity [13, 15]. The morphine-6 glucuronide and morphine-3 glucuronide metabolites of morphine can accumulate in renal dysfunction and cause respiratory depression, sedation, nausea, vomiting, and neuroexcitation (allodynia, myoclonus, seizures) [15]. The hydromorphone metabolite hydromorphone-3 glucuronide can also cause neuroexcitation if accumulation occurs [15]. In patients with renal impairment, codeine can cause hypotension, respiratory depression, and narcolepsy [15]. Normeperidine, the neurotoxic metabolite of meperidine, is renally cleared and has a longer elimination half-life than the parent drug (3 h vs. 15–30 h) [13]. Normeperidine can accumulate in renal dysfunction, causing toxicity [13].

Due to the increased risk of toxicity, the opioids morphine, codeine, and hydromorphone are not recommended for patients with renal failure [15]. Limited information is available regarding the use of buprenorphine, oxycodone, oxymorphone, and tapentadol in renal failure. However, fentanyl and methadone, which are metabolized to inactive metabolites, may be preferred in patients with renal dysfunction to minimize the risk of accumulation [13, 15]. Methadone's inactive metabolites are excreted in the feces and thus are not expected to accumulate in patients with renal dysfunction [13]. Extended-release tramadol is contraindicated in severe renal impairment [15]. Because most opioids or their metabolites are renally excreted, opioid therapy is best initiated at low doses and titrated slowly [15]. Additionally, patients should be carefully monitored for supratherapeutic drug concentrations and signs and symptoms of adverse effects [15].

Patients with Hepatic Impairment

When patients have hepatic impairment, glucuronidation is impacted less than CYP-mediated metabolism [15]. Therefore, opioids such as morphine, hydromorphone, and oxymorphone, which are metabolized by glucuronidation rather than CYP-enzymes, may be preferable, although they are still impacted to some extent by hepatic impairment [15]. While fentanyl is metabolized by CYP3A4, it is still recommended for use in patients with hepatic failure [15]. Hydromorphone, morphine, oxycodone, and methadone are cautiously recommended [15]. The use of codeine, oxymorphone, and tramadol is not recommended in patients with hepatic failure [15]. Limited information is available regarding the use of buprenorphine, hydrocodone, and tapentadol in patients with hepatic failure [15].

In patients with moderate hepatic impairment, hydromorphone exhibits mean and maximum plasma concentrations four times greater than those in patients without hepatic dysfunction [15]. Oxymorphone is contraindicated in patients with moderate to severe hepatic dysfunction because bioavailability may be increased 1.6- to 12.2-fold in these patients [15]. Opioids metabolized by CYP enzymes are not necessarily contraindicated in patients with liver impairment; fentanyl and methadone, for example, are both metabolized by CYP enzymes but less affected by hepatic impairment than other opioids [15].

Summary

Appropriate pain management in the elderly requires an understanding of the physiologic changes that occur with aging and their impact on drug pharmacokinetics and pharmacodynamics.

References

1. Gibson SJ. In: Dostrovsk JO, Carr DB, Kaltenzburg M, editors. Proceedings of the 10th world congress on pain, progress in pain research and management. Vol. 24. Seattle, WA: IASP Press; 2003. p. 767–90.
2. Kaye AD, Baluch A, Scott JT. Pain management in the elderly population: a review. Ochsner J. 2010;10:179–87.
3. Davis MP, Srivastava M. Demographics, assessment and management of pain in the elderly. Drugs Aging. 2003;20(1):23–57.
4. Morrone FB, Schroeter G, Petitembert AP, et al. Potential interactions of central nervous system drugs used in the elderly population. BJP. 2009;45(2):227–33.
5. Holmgaar R, Benfeldt E, Sorensen JA, et al. Chronological age affects the permeation of fentanyl through human skin in vitro. Skin Pharmacol Physiol. 2013;26:155–9.
6. Klotz U. Pharmacokinetics and drug metabolism in the elderly. Drug Metab Rev. 2009;41(2):67–76.
7. Turnheim K. When drug therapy gets old: pharmacokinetics and pharmacodynamics in the elderly. Exp Gerontol. 2003;38:843–53.
8. Mercadante S, Arcuri E. Pharmacological management of cancer pain in the elderly. Drugs Aging. 2007;24(9):761–76.

9. Rowland M, Tozer TN. Clinical pharmacokinetics concepts and applications. 3rd ed. Philadelphia: Lippincott Williams & Williams; 1995.
10. Duragesic Prescribing Information. http://www.duragesic.com/prescribing-information.html. Accessed 27 Sept 2013.
11. Scully C. Drug effects on salivary glands: dry mouth. Oral Dis. 2003;9:165–76.
12. Reisner L. Pharmacological management of persistent pain in older persons. J Pain. 2011;12(3):S21–9.
13. Trescot AM, Datta S, Lee M, et al. Opioid pharmacology. Pain Physician. 2008;11:S133–53.
14. Cavalieri TA. Management of pain in older adults. JAOA. 2005;105(3):S12–7.
15. Smith H, Bruckenthal P. Implications of opioid analgesia for medically complicated patients. Drugs Aging. 2010;27(5):417–33.
16. The American Geriatrics Society 2015 Beers Criteria Update Expert Panel. American geriatrics society 2015 updated beers criteria for potentially inappropriate medication use in older adults. J Am Geriatr Soc. 2015;63(11):2227–46.
17. Koper D, Kamenski G, Flamm M, et al. Frequency of medication errors in primary care patients with polypharmacy. Fam Pract. 2013;30:313–9.
18. Zhao J, Xin X, Xie G, et al. Molecular and cellular mechanisms of the age-dependency of opioid analgesia and tolerance. Mol Pain. 2012;10(38):1–12.
19. Buntin-Mushock C, Phillip L, Moriyama K, et al. Age-dependent opioid escalation in chronic pain patients. Anesth Analg. 2005;100(6):1740–5.
20. Kugler JP, Hustead T. Hyponatremia and hypernatremia in the elderly. Am Fam Physician. 2000;61(12):3623–30.
21. Lea M, Rognan SE, Koristovic R, et al. Severity and management of drug-drug interactions in acute geriatric patients. Drugs Aging. 2013;30:721–7.
22. McPherson ML. Frequent pharmacological interactions. In: Oxford American handbook of hospice and palliative medicine. New York: Oxford UP; 2011. p. 314–32. Print.
23. Boyer EW, Shannon M. The serotonin syndrome. N Engl J Med. 2005;352(11):1112–20.
24. Liu WQ, Kanungo A, Toth C. Equivalency of tricyclic antidepressants in open-label neuropathic pain study. Acta Neurol Scand. 2013;129(2):132–41.
25. U.S. Food and Drug Administration. FDA News Release: Xanodyne agrees to withdraw propoxyphene from the U.S. market. Nov. 19, 2010. http://www.fda.gov/NewsEvents/Newsroom/PressAnnouncements/ucm234350.htm. Accessed 28 Sept 2013.
26. U.S. Food and Drug Administration. Recent FDA actions on NSAIDs. FDA patient safety news: show #40 2005. http://www.accessdata.fda.gov/scripts/cdrh/cfdocs/psn/printer.cfm?id=328. Accessed 28 Sept 2013.
27. Butrans Prescribing Information. http://app.purduepharma.com/xmlpublishing/pi.aspx?id=b. Accessed 27 Sept 2013.
28. McPherson ML, Cimino NM. Topical NSAID formulations. Pain Med. 2013;14:S25–9.
29. Abstral Prescribing Information. http://dailymed.nlm.nih.gov/dailymed/lookup.cfm?setid=f969e2bc-6297-4e29-89d3-a3685a2c7c6b. Accessed 28 Sept 2013.
30. Actiq Prescribing Information. http://dailymed.nlm.nih.gov/dailymed/lookup.cfm?setid=90b94524-f913-48b3-3771-7b2fcffd888a. Accessed 28 Sept 2013.
31. Lazanda Prescribing Information. http://dailymed.nlm.nih.gov/dailymed/lookup.cfm?setid=39531d0c-db12-4627-81c9-6563076b637b. Accessed 28 Sept 2013.
32. Subsys Prescribing Information. http://dailymed.nlm.nih.gov/dailymed/lookup.cfm?setid=18a413e9-11e0-4a8f-86c0-d33b37b7b771. Accessed 28 Sept 2013.

Specific Conditions Causing Persistent Pain in Older Adults

Charles E. Argoff, Ravneet Bhullar, and Katherine Galluzzi

Introduction

The observation that there may be more people over the age of 65 alive today than the total number who have ever reached that age is a stunning testament to our success at increasing longevity. However, with increasing numbers of elders comes the challenge of maintaining their quality of life. It is a fact of aging that chronic medical conditions will accrue, some of which may progress to chronic pain states. Persistent pain has become a chronic disease itself, like diabetes or hypertension.

Among the diagnoses that cause persistent pain are diabetes mellitus, cancer, fibromyalgia, osteoarthritis, polymyalgia rheumatica, postherpetic neuralgia, poststroke pain, and spinal stenosis. Older adults undergo surgery for cancer, coronary heart disease, and other acute problems; they also undergo elective surgical procedures such as joint replacement with greater frequency than younger persons. It is now clear that inadequately treated acute postsurgical pain may progress to become persistent pain.

Older individuals may have various coexisting sources of pain which present the clinical challenge of how to best manage several etiologies for pain at a time when the use of pharmacologic agents is constrained by comorbid disease states and/or inevitable age-related physiologic changes. This chapter will provide a framework for addressing specific chronic pain conditions. Careful history, physical examination, and formal pain assessment are the cornerstones for developing a treatment plan of care that incorporates focused, cost-effective diagnostic testing and evidence-based best practices for treatment. Multimodal treatment interventions will be suggested, with the goal of reducing persistent pain and increasing quality of life into old age.

C. E. Argoff (✉)
Albany Medical College, Albany, NY, USA

R. Bhullar
Albany Medical Center, Department of Anesthesiology, Albany, NY, USA

K. Galluzzi
Philadelphia College of Osteopathic Medicine, Philadelphia, PA, USA

Overview

Discussion of persistent pain must consider the basic pathophysiology of aging. Age-related physiologic changes in body habitus (increased fat to lean ratio), joint and vertebral mobility (arthritis, chondrocalcinosis), energy level (metabolic, endocrine changes), and gait and balance (neuropathy, deconditioning) influence one's level of activity. Acquired disease negatively impacts the ability to withstand stress of illness and/or surgery. These factors combine to constitute one's overall level of health and function, which in turn may predict one's predisposition to developing one or more painful conditions.

Age-related physiologic changes result in altered pharmacokinetics. While changes in gastric pH cause minimal effect on drug absorption, there are more significant changes in drug distribution, altered renal and hepatic metabolism, and decreased excretion. Altered pharmacokinetics must guide pharmaceutical prescribing: there are some analgesic medications that are rarely appropriate for geriatric use.

The American Geriatric Society (AGS [1]) 2012 Beer's Criteria Update Expert Panel has expanded recommendations to include medications that are potentially inappropriate to be used in specific disease states as well as drugs to be used either with caution or completely avoided. Updated guidelines by the AGS Panel on Pharmacological Management of Persistent Pain (2009 [2]) remain as a valuable resource (see Table 1) for a concise review of age-related physiologic changes and their effect on analgesic pharmacologic choices for older individuals.

Additionally, experts have identified other specific medications to completely avoid or use only with caution in older adults. The nonsteriodal anti-inflammatory drugs (NSAIDs) indomethacin, ketorolac, naproxen, oxaprozin, and piroxicam, due to their diminished renal excretion in older adults, increase the risk of bleeding as well as renal and cardiotoxicity and should therefore be avoided. Certain opioid analgesics (pentazocine, propoxyphene, and meperidine) and skeletal muscle relaxants (carisoprodol, cyclobenzaprine, methocarbamol, and chlorzoxazone) have adverse effects and should be avoided. The risks of prescribing these drugs outweigh the potential analgesic benefits in older individuals [3].

Many pain syndromes respond well to nonpharmacologic therapies. For older adults, the attempt to find a suitable alternative to a medication is a management tenet. Even if medication is an indicated, important, or essential treatment option, nonpharmacologic therapies should be sought and integrated as part of a multimodal treatment plan. Clinicians should bear in mind the fact that all treatments, including the decision not to treat, have risks as well as benefits.

Table 1 *Pharmacologic changes with aging.* There may be age-associated differences in the effectiveness, sensitivity, toxicity, and pharmacokinetics or pharmacodynamics of certain drugs in older patients (>65 years). The following table summarizes some potential changes that may occur during normal aging and affect patients' responses to analgesics

Pharmacology	Change with normal aging	Common disease effects
Liver metabolism	Oxidation is variable and may decrease resulting in prolonged drug half-life	Cirrhosis, hepatitis, and tumors may disrupt oxidation but not usually conjugation
	Conjugation is usually preserved	
	First-pass effect usually unchanged	
	Genetic enzyme polymorphisms may affect some cytochrome enzymes	
Renal excretion	GFR decreases with advancing age, resulting in decreased excretion	Chronic kidney disease may predispose further to renal toxicity
Transdermal absorption	Few changes in absorption based on age may be related to patch technology used	Temperature and other specific patch characteristics may affect absorption
GI absorption or function	Slowing of GI transit time (may prolong effects of continuous-release enteral drugs)	Disorders that alter gastric pH and surgically altered anatomy may reduce absorption of some drugs
	Enhanced opioid-related bowel dysmotility	
Active metabolites	Reduced renal clearance will prolong effects of metabolites	Renal disease increase in half-life
Anticholinergic side effects	Increased confusion, constipation, incontinence, movement disorders	Enhanced by neurological disease processes
Distribution	Increased fat to lean body weight ratio may increase volume of distribution for fat-soluble drugs	Aging and obesity may result in longer effective drug half-life

Adapted from: American Geriatrics Society Panel on the Pharmacological Management of Persistent Pain in Older Persons [2]

Clinical Presentation: General Considerations

The presentation of an older adult with a painful condition varies considerably based on that person's experience and understanding of the pain. Geriatric clinicians cite the tendency of some older patients to underreport painful symptoms. The reasons for this are many and include fear of the meaning of the pain, fear of painful diagnostic procedures, fear of being perceived as a complainer, or fear of not being heard or believed. A related concern is the fear that there may be nothing that can or will be done to ameliorate the pain, thus producing a form of therapeutic nihilism.

Many studies have examined the effects of gender and age on pain. In general, younger women exhibit lower pain thresholds and experience more severe pain than age-matched men exposed to similar noxious stimuli; they also have higher rates of certain pain states such as osteoarthritis, migraines, and fibromyalgia. While the reason for this is unclear, it has been postulated that hormonal differences may play a part. Decreased estrogen postmenopause and, to a lesser extent, diminishing levels of testosterone in older men may account for the observation that response to pain tends to be similar between older women and men. It has also been observed that the pain response is not blunted with age but may in fact increase, especially for men – which may further explain why the pain response in older adults shows less gender difference.

Numerous barriers exist regarding the management of pain in older patients. Among older persons, cultural barriers, fears about the possibility of addiction, and sensory and cognitive impairments all have an impact on achieving optimal pain relief. Clinicians face further difficulties in managing older patients with pain including lack of recognition of pain, lack of adequate pain management training, and limited time in busy office settings. Mindful of these challenges, clinicians caring for older individuals must be especially vigilant in recognizing nonverbal clues or physical signals that suggest that the patient is withholding information about pain. Since older adults with cognitive or verbal impairment may be unable to self-report, clinicians should consult with their caregiver(s) to gather information about the pain, specifically evaluating exacerbating and alleviating factors, the duration and quality of the pain, and its impact on function (Kerr) [4].

There are a number of assessment tools for pain, including but not limited to:

- Brief Pain Inventory
- Faces Scales
- Functional Pain Scale (FPS)
- Iowa Pain Thermometer
- Numeric Pain Intensity Scales
- Short Form-McGill Pain Questionnaire (SF-MPQ)
- Verbal Descriptor Scale
- Visual Analogue Scale

In every case, clinicians should obtain a thorough pain assessment, including precipitating, exacerbating, and mitigating factors. Patients and/or caregivers should be asked to rate the pain; keeping a pain diary may help pinpoint causative factors as well as identify potential coping mechanisms.

The fundamental goals of clinical assessment of pain are to:

- Achieve diagnosis of pain.
- Identify and treat underlying causes of neuropathy.
- Identify and treat comorbid conditions.
- Evaluate psychosocial factors.
- Evaluate functional status (activity levels).
- Set goals.
- Develop a targeted treatment plan.
- Determine whether a consultation is needed.

In addition to the above goals, a crucial first step in diagnosis and treatment of pain is to acknowledge to the patient that he or she is experiencing pain and that the pain is real. A pain-specific history; thorough physical exam with pain-specific sensory evaluation; musculoskeletal, myofascial, and neurologic assessment; and a psychological evaluation are basic required elements.

Specific chronic pain-causing conditions to be reviewed in this chapter are grouped according to three main categories:

- Disease states:
  - Cancer
    - Painful metastases and bone pain
    - Radiation fibrosis and chemotherapy-induced painful neuropathy
  - Diabetes mellitus
    - Painful diabetic peripheral neuropathy
  - Herpes zoster
    - Acute infection
    - Postherpetic neuralgia
  - Polymyalgia rheumatica
- Degenerative conditions:
  - Osteoarthritis
  - Spinal stenosis
  - Compression fractures
  - Contractures and pressure ulcers
  - Low back pain
    - Muscle strain/sprain
    - Sciatica
    - Herniated disk
    - Piriformis syndrome
- Abnormal central processing disorders:
  - Fibromyalgia
  - Persistent postoperative pain syndromes
  - Central poststroke pain

Although each of these pain states will be discussed separately, they share common characteristics, and many, if not all, fall under more than one topic area. For example, painful diabetic peripheral neuropathy and postherpetic neuralgia are disease-induced painful states and also examples of peripheral and central sensitization. An attempt to draw parallels between these diagnostic categories will be made; it is our hope that the reader will gain a greater appreciation of the commonalities that exist among patterns of pain in older adults.

Diseases Resulting in Persistent Pain

Both acquired and infectious diseases can be the origin of persistent pain states. Cancer causes chronic pain due to tumor burden and metastasis and as a consequence of treatment, such as surgery, radiation, and/or chemotherapy. Cancer treatments may cause neuronal destruction which results in neuropathic pain. Directly or indirectly, the pain of cancer may be nociceptive, neuropathic, or mixed. Bennett et al. [5] note that it is important to distinguish between neuropathic cancer pain (neuropathic pain caused directly by cancer) and neuropathic pain in a cancer patient (caused by cancer treatment or comorbid disease). Some cancer survivors defeat malignancy but acquire the condition of persistent pain.

Diabetes mellitus, which is becoming a worldwide epidemic, causes painful diabetic peripheral neuropathy (PDPN); herpes zoster ("shingles") – the reactivation of latent varicella zoster virus – causes both acute pain and postherpetic neuralgia (PHN) which is defined as pain that persists after the rash of acute infection has healed. PDPN and PHN share a common pathologic denominator: development of abnormal central pain processing (painful neuropathy) caused by disease-related destruction of neuronal tissue.

The International Association for the Study of Pain Neuropathic Pain Special Interest Group (NeuPSIG) has defined criteria for diagnosis of neuropathic pain which may assist clinicians in assessment of patients. The NeuPSIG criteria include:

1. Pain distribution is neuroanatomically plausible.
2. History is suggestive of relevant lesion or disease.
3. Negative or positive sensory signs within innervation's territory of lesion are present.
4. A diagnostic test confirms lesion or disease.

When evaluating a patient with a potential disease-induced form of pain, these criteria can help differentiate nociceptive from neuropathic types of pain and thus guide treatment choices.

Cancer Pain

The prevalence of pain in the adult cancer population is estimated at 41%, while those with advanced cancer have pain prevalence rates of 75%, with a range of 50–100%. There is little pain data for cancer survivors, who represent a large and growing group of patients, especially among the older adult population. There are numerous potential etiologies for cancer pain, among them:

- Tumor burden
- Diagnostic procedures
- Postoperative
- Radiation
- Chemotherapy
- Hormonal
- Metastasis
- Infection

Cancer pain can be the direct result of the malignancy or the result of treatment and is characterized by nociceptive (bone pain), visceral (hepatic distention, malignant bowel obstruction), neuropathic (leptomeningeal metastases, cranial neuralgia, radiculopathy, paraneoplastic), or mixed (caused by two or more etiologies). Patients with cancer may also experience psychological or existential pain, especially those for whom the cancer represents a terminal illness. For these patients, palliative medicine can provide symptom management and supportive care that involves an interdisciplinary team including medical, nursing, social work, and pastoral counseling services.

The goals of care for patients with cancer pain are to:

- Prevent discomfort when possible.
- Reduce baseline pain as much as possible.
  - Long-acting (extended or controlled release) analgesics
  - Adjuvant medications
  - Therapeutic blocks
- Aggressively treat episodes of breakthrough pain.
  - Acute, transient, and worsening
  - Short-acting (immediate-release) analgesics

The presentation of new pain in a patient with a history of cancer should prompt a thorough evaluation for cancer recurrence or metastasis. Types of cancer that typically metastasize to osseous structures include lung, breast, and prostate, but thyroid and renal carcinomas also spread to bone. Bony metastasis is difficult to cure since it generally is not amenable to surgery; it can lead to significant complications such as pathologic fractures, spinal cord and nerve compression, as well as intractable pain. The pain of bone metastasis is due to prostaglandin release so anti-inflammatory medications (NSAIDs, steroids) may be useful. Steroids are also useful for reducing edema in tumor and surrounding nerve tissue, and they are standard emergency treatment for suspected malignant spinal cord compression, followed by surgery if indicated. Treatments for pain from bone metastasis are:

- Systemic analgesics
- Glucocorticoids
- Intrathecal analgesics
- Radiation
  - External beam, radiopharmaceuticals
- Ablation
  - Radiofrequency and cryoablation
- Bisphosphonates
- Chemotherapeutic agents
- RANKL-RANK inhibitors (denosumab)
- Hormonal therapies
- Interventional procedures (kyphoplasty, vertebroplasty)
- Surgery

Neuropathic pain from tumor compression or nerve destruction may respond to anticonvulsants (gabapentin, pregabalin, carbamazepine, sodium valproate, phenytoin), tricyclic antidepressants (nortriptyline, desipramine, imipramine), or serotonin-norepinephrine reuptake inhibitors (duloxetine, venlafaxine). Table 6 lists medications for painful diabetic peripheral neuropathy which may also be beneficial treatment options for cancer-related neuropathic pain.

Colon cancer and other gastrointestinal malignancies typically metastasize to the liver. The pain associated with GI tumor is visceral pain; ascites and increased abdominal distension may also cause discomfort. First-line treatment options include diuretics and analgesics. In patients in whom diuretic therapy fails, paracentesis to reduce ascites is a valuable comfort measure. Patients with malignant bowel obstruction may require nasogastric suction to decrease abdominal distension. If surgery is not an option, corticosteroids (dexamethasone) may relieve the obstruction. Failing this, complete bowel rest is needed; treatment of nausea may respond to metoclopramide or antiemetics. Glycopyrrolate, haloperidol, and hyoscyamine are helpful to reduce nausea and lessen GI secretions. In severe cases, subcutaneously administered octreotide may quiet the bowel, reduce secretions, and relieve pain. Despite these measures, opioid analgesics are frequently required to reduce visceral pain.

Brain metastasis or primary brain tumors, in addition to causing cognitive and neurologic deficits (such as changes in vision), cause cephalgia. Corticosteroids reduce intracranial swelling and inflammation and provide analgesia.

While non-opioid and adjunctive analgesics may be helpful, for patients with diffuse metastasis or advanced disease and for those with mixed nociceptive and neuropathic cancer pain, opioid analgesics are the mainstay of treatment. Opioids are potent mu, kappa, and delta (and many subtype) receptor agonists with little or no ceiling effect; that is, they maintain efficacy with dose escalation, which will be needed due to the development of opioid tolerance. Multiple formulations are available (pill, liquid, injectable, transdermal, rectal, buccal film) and useful for those who have difficulty swallowing and/or are unable to take medications on a precise schedule.

Table 2 classifies types of opioids as naturally occurring, synthetic, or semisynthetic.

Table 3 suggests starting doses for adults weighing over 50 Kilograms.

Also please refer to the discussion of morphine and hydromorphone metabolism in the section on persistent postsurgical pain in this chapter for information about renal dosing.

Several opioid analgesics, including morphine and oxycodone, are available in short-acting, immediate-release (IR), long-acting, controlled release (CR), and extended release (ER) formulations. A goal of care for cancer pain is to provide a baseline level of comfort through the use of a long-acting preparation. Breakthrough pain, defined as pain occurring either episodically or incident to certain situations (like dressing changes or movement) that is not controlled by long-acting opioid, requires an immediate-release opioid on an as-needed basis (see Tables 4 and 5).

Table 2 Classification of opioid analgesics

Naturally occurring opioids	Opium, morphine, codeine, thebaine
Semisynthetic opioids	Heroin, oxycodone, hydrocodone, oxymorphone, hydromorphone
Synthetic	Methadone, meperidine, fentanyl, levorphanol, propoxyphene
Mixed antagonists	Buprenorphine, nalbuphine, pentazocine, butorphanol
Antagonists	Naltrexone, naloxone, nalmefene
Novel agents	Tramadol, tramadol extended release, tapentadol

Kroenke et al. [12]

Table 3 Oral opioid dosing chart

Codeine	50–60 mg	Q 3–4 h
Oxycodone	5–10 mg	Q 3–4 h
Morphine	10–30 mg	Q 3–4 h
Hydromorphone	2–6 mg	Q 3–4 h
Oxymorphone	10–20 mg	Q 4–6 h
Tramadol	50–100 mg	Q 4–6 h
Tapentadol	50–100 mg	Q 4–6 h

Galvagno et al. [13]. Nucynta [package insert]. Titusville, NJ: PriCara, Division of Ortho-McNeil Janssen Pharmaceuticals, Inc.; 2008.

Table 4 Short-acting opioids – equianalgesic doses

Hydrocodone	30 mg
Oxycodone	30 mg
Codeine	120 mg
Morphine	30 mg
Hydromorphone	7.5 mg
Oxymorphone	10 mg
Tapentadol	50 mg
Tramadol	50 mg

Adapted from: Argoff and Silvershein [14]

Table 5 Long-acting opioids – equianalgesic doses

Morphine controlled release	90–120 mg every 12 h
Morphine extended release	180–240 mg every 24 h
Oxycodone extended release	40 mg every 12 h
Methadone	20 mg every 12 h
Fentanyl patch	25 mcgm every 72 h
Oxymorphone extended release	30–40 every 12 h
Tramadol extended release	100 mg

Adapted from: Argoff and Silvershein [14]

For those who are no longer able to swallow liquids, opioids may be administered either intravenously (e.g., PCA pump) or subcutaneously, either through bolus or continuous infusion, or via intrathecal or epidural routes of administration.

Anticancer treatments that cause pain include:

- Surgery
  - Post-surgery syndromes, phantom pain
- Radiation
  - Plexopathies
- Chemotherapy
  - Painful neuropathy, bony complications of long-term steroids
- Hormonal
  - Compression fractures, arthralgia (aromatase inhibitors)

Post-chemotherapy pain is frequently neuropathic and may respond to anticonvulsant, tricyclic antidepressant, or opioid analgesics. Radiation fibrosis, a common consequence of radiation therapy for cancer, can result in destruction of lymphatic or connective tissue with the sequela of edema, pleuritis, or painful contractures. Radiation can also cause proctitis, enteritis, nephropathy, and gastrointestinal or cutaneous ulcers. Treatments should be directed, when possible, at reducing or minimizing the extent of radiation injury, and when necessary, utilizing the pain armamentarium already described.

It is especially important to seek multimodal therapy for patients experiencing cancer pain. Persons with serious or terminal illness experience existential pain which may amplify physical discomfort. A multimodal approach may utilize medications, nonpharmacologic options, as well as complementary and alternative therapies to achieve adequate pain control and enhanced quality of life; members of an interdisciplinary team of providers, including physicians, advanced practice nurses or physician assistants, social workers, and pastoral counselors, are a valuable resource.

For intractable pain at the end of life, palliative (terminal) sedation may be the only alternative, which includes use of medications such as lorazepam, midazolam, ketamine, or propofol. Palliative sedation for intractable pain requires the support of both the patient's family/caregivers and the medical team, who recognize that all possible etiologies and treatment options have been exhausted. Clinicians must educate patients and families regarding their goals and the outcomes, and in this instance, an interdisciplinary team approach is crucial [6].

Painful Diabetic Peripheral Neuropathy

The incidence of painful diabetic peripheral neuropathy (PDPN) is likely to increase as the population ages and as the numbers of people with diabetes mellitus increase. Next to low back-associated neuropathic pain, PDPN is the most common cause of neuropathic pain. Current estimates of the prevalence of PDPN among adults with diabetes range from 26% to 47% [7].

Diabetic peripheral neuropathy has a characteristic pattern of signs and symptoms; it begins as paresthesia or dysesthesia in a "stocking-glove" distribution, especially in the feet and lower legs, which can progress to frank neuropathic pain. The pain is typically described as burning, searing, or numbness, although patients may use any of the following descriptors, among others:

- Tingling
- Crawling
- Shooting
- Stabbing
- Electrical
- Shock-like

The discomfort may be severe enough to disrupt sleep and can have a negative effect on quality of life in patients who are faced with both treatment challenges and further complications of diabetes. Currently there is no effective "cure" for PDPN, and efforts must be directed at prevention through good glycemic control.

Evaluation of patients complaining of PDPN should include somatosensory function, including vibration, thermal, light touch, and pain perception, as well as inspection, palpation, and use of an appropriate pain scale, such as the Brief Pain Inventory, short form. Other tools specifically designed to assess neuropathic pain include:

- Neuropathic Pain Scale (NPS) [8]
  - Expert opinion; 10 items
- Distinctions: deep and surface pain; sensation and unpleasantness
- Neuropathic Pain Questionnaire (NPQ) [9]
  - Empirically derived; 10 items
- Neuropathic Pain Symptom Inventory (NPSI) [10]
  - Empirically derived; 12 items
- Distinctions: spontaneous pain, evoked pain, paroxysms, paresthesias

The 10 g monofilament is a useful physical exam tool for evaluating sensory loss. Other diagnostic tests may include nerve conduction velocity or nerve biopsy. However, as suggested by the NeuPSIG, in most cases, a clinical diagnosis can be made through careful history and physical, assessment of distribution and pattern of pain, and evaluation of sensory and trophic changes in the painful region(s) of an individual who has been diagnosed with diabetes mellitus.

Goals of care for patients with painful diabetic peripheral neuropathy are to:

- Prevent further nerve destruction through good glycemic control
- Provide relief from paresthesias, dysesthesias, or frank pain
- Maintain physical function, adequate sleep, and improve quality of life

Beyond achieving glycemic control, treatment for PDPN is palliative and symptom-oriented. Alpha-2 delta ligands, topical analgesics, opioids, tricyclic antidepressants, and serotonin-norepinephrine reuptake inhibitors have FDA approval for treatment of PDPN. Table 6 lists pharmacologic treatment options.

Nonpharmacologic treatment options for PDPN include those recommended for any chronic painful condition: lifestyle modification (stress reduction, exercise), interferential therapy, cognitive behavioral therapy (CBT), TENS units, heat and/or cold application, osteopathic and other manual medicine techniques, and massage and acupuncture.

A detailed history may help to determine which (or combination) of the above therapies will be of most benefit. Many PDPN sufferers complain that the pain is intolerable at night and causes them to lose sleep, while during the day, it is less annoying. These individuals may benefit most from an appropriate dose of a relatively sedating medication at bedtime, such as pregabalin or nortriptyline combined with CBT techniques to assist with falling and remaining asleep. While it may not be possible to obtain complete relief, PDPN can often be effectively managed with a combination of good glycemic control, appropriate pharmacologic agent(s), and nonpharmacologic interventions aimed at preserving function and providing the best possible quality of life.

Table 6 Pharmacologic treatments for PDPN

Pharmacologic class	Individual agent(s)
Selective serotonin-norepinephrine inhibitors (SNRIs)	Duloxetine[a], venlafaxine
$\alpha_2\delta$ ligands (modulate voltage-gated calcium channels – synaptic release of several neurotransmitters, e.g., glutamate)	Pregabalin[a], gabapentin
Tricyclic antidepressants (TCAs) (inhibit reuptake of serotonin and norepinephrine)	Secondary: desipramine Tertiary: *amitriptyline (see below)*
Opioids (Bind to μ-opioid receptors)	Tramadol, oxycodone CR, morphine, methadone, levorphanol, hydromorphone, tapentadol ER[a]
Topical agents	Capsaicin, lidocaine patch
Agents to avoid (never use)	*Meperidine (metabolite normeperidine – central nervous system toxicity)* *NSAIDs (increased risk of bleeding, GI upset, cardio- or cerebrovascular events)* *Acetaminophen (hepatotoxicity)* *Amitriptyline (pts >60 yrs)* *Vit B_6 (potential for neurotoxicity)* *Pentazocine (CNS toxicity {mixed agonist-antagonist})*

[a]FDA-approved; http://www.fda.gov/default.htm

Herpes Zoster/Postherpetic Neuralgia

Varicella zoster virus (VZV) is a viral pathogen that leads two lives: first as chicken pox and later as herpes zoster or "shingles." Following acute infection (chicken pox), VZV recedes to dormancy in the dorsal root ganglia. When the affected individual's cell-mediated immunity drops below a threshold, zoster recrudesces to manifest as a painful dermatomal rash. The neuropathic pain of shingles is acute and may persist or develop after the rash has healed: postherpetic neuralgia (PHN). Acute zoster pain is described as mild to severe burning, itching, or tingling, typically present prior to the development of the rash. It has been noted that the more extensive the rash and severe the acute pain, the more intense the development of postherpetic neuralgia, due to the destruction of neuronal tissue by the varicella zoster virus.

The lifetime incidence of herpes zoster infection is estimated to be about one in five. While it is clear that prevention of herpes zoster infection by immunization (Shingrix, Zostavax) is a best clinical practice, many individuals will nevertheless experience an episode of shingles. Early recognition of the prodrome to herpes zoster is vital since this enables clinicians to intervene in a timely fashion to reduce the burden of illness.

Although the systemic symptoms are usually mild, zoster may be accompanied by fever and malaise, and if inadequately treated, it can progress to systemic complications, noted below. Prior to the development of an erythematous vesicular rash, patients may complain of pain in a characteristic pattern of one or two dermatomes that manifests as burning, itching, or tingling. The pain may mimic headache, brachial neuritis, cardiac or abdominal pain, or sciatica. Less commonly, zoster can occur without a rash. Antiviral medication, e.g., acyclovir, should be instituted at the earliest sign of infection in an attempt to reduce the neuronal destruction caused by the virus and potentially to avoid development of postherpetic neuralgia. Early treatment may also reduce the risk for complications, which may be neurologic (motor neuropathy, cranial palsy, encephalitis, transverse myelitis, or postzoster stroke syndromes), cutaneous (bacterial superinfection, scarring, disfigurement), ophthalmic (stromal keratitis, iritis, retinitis, visual impairment, episcleritis, or keratopathy), or visceral (pneumonitis, hepatitis, or encephalitis).

Severity and extent of the shingles rash, advanced age, and increased debility strongly correlate with the potential for PHN. In addition to antiviral medication, acute control of pain with an appropriate analgesic is essential.

The primary goals of care for herpes zoster are to:

- Shorten the course of illness
- Provide adequate analgesia
- Prevent complications
- Prevent the development of PHN

Antiviral medication (acyclovir and its derivatives: famciclovir, valacyclovir, or penciclovir) should be initiated at the first sign of acute herpes zoster infection, ideally within the first 72 h of infection. The earlier the antiviral is started, the more effective in shortening the course of illness and reducing or preventing PHN.

Corticosteroid treatment for acute zoster infection is controversial. Some treatment studies (e.g., prednisone 40–60 mg daily for 1 week followed by a rapid taper) show decreased incidence of the development of PHN, while others have failed to show benefit. The potential for adverse effects of corticosteroids (salt and water retention, hyperglycemia, and central nervous system effects) must be weighed against the potential, theoretical reduction of neuronal destruction. In general, most clinicians reserve treatment with corticosteroids for cases of severe, complicated, or extensive infection.

Analgesic agents for reduction of pain in acute herpes zoster include opioid and non-opioid analgesics, tricyclic antidepressants, and anticonvulsants. Analgesic treatment should begin as early as possible, as with antiviral medications.

Table 7 shows management strategies for acute herpes zoster.

Pain that persists after resolution of rash (PHN) will require continued treatment and may have improved pain control using one or more available agents (Table 8).

As with all forms of chronic pain, PHN may best respond to a choice of multimodal therapies that include both pharmacologic and nonpharmacologic options.

Polymyalgia Rheumatica

Polymyalgia rheumatic (PMR) is an inflammatory condition that causes pain in the neck, shoulders, and pelvic girdle of people over the age of 50, usually Caucasian women. PMR can present as aching, unremitting pain in the shoulders and neck, sometimes involving the pelvis/hips, stiffness, and unexplained weight loss. The exact etiology of PMR is unclear, but there does seem to be a seasonal prevalence, and it is likely that there are genetic determinants that may predispose to its development.

Table 7 Management strategies for acute herpes zoster

Medication	Whom to treat	Limitations
Oral antivirals	Patients with zoster rash	Use within 72 h of rash onset
IV acyclovir	Selective use in immunosuppressed patients or those with CNS disease	May use after 72 h in immunosuppressed
Oral corticosteroids	Adjunctive therapy for patients with moderate to severe pain (controversial)	Use with caution in patients with underlying illnesses
Aspirin, NSAIDs, antihistamines, calamine, silver sulfadiazine	Patients with minor pain or itching	May not provide adequate pain relief
Opioids	Patients with moderate to severe pain	Significant side effects, potential for addiction

Table 8 Treatment of postherpetic neuralgia

Medication	Pain response and adverse event profile
Gabapentin, pregabalin[a,b]	33% reduction with gabapentin; 63% significant pain reduction with pregabalin. Adverse events include somnolence, dizziness, and peripheral edema
Tricyclic antidepressants[c]	47–67% of patients report at least moderate pain relief. Adverse events: sedation, confusion, urinary retention, dry mouth, postural hypotension, arrhythmia
Opioid analgesics[d,e]	38–58% of patients report pain relief. Adverse events: constipation, nausea, loss of appetite, dizziness, and drowsiness
Lidocaine patch 5%[f]	60% efficacy (i.e., at least moderate pain relief). No systemic adverse events, but local reactions include erythema and skin rash
Topical Capsaicin 8% patch[g,h]	Only one application needed. Requires pretreatment with topical local anesthetic
Opioids	Patients with moderate to severe pain

Gabapentin, pregabalin, lidocaine patch 5%, and topical capsaicin are FDA approved for the treatment of PHN
[a]Rowbotham et al. [15]
[b]Dworkin et al. [16]
[c]Pappagallo and Haldey [17]
[d]Watson and Babul [18]
[e]Raja et al. [19]
[f]Davies and Galer [20]
[g]Watson et al. [21]
[h]Derry et al. [22]

PMR is disproportionately associated with giant cell arteritis (GCA) which is an inflammation of vascular endothelium characterized as a granulomatous vasculitis that affects the aorta and other major blood vessels. One form of GCA, temporal arteritis, if inadequately treated, can lead to vision loss.

PMR can be difficult to differentiate from other rheumatological conditions such as rheumatoid arthritis or ankylosing spondylitis. In April of 2012, the American College of Rheumatology (ACR) and the European Union League Against Rheumatism (EULAR) have established criteria for the diagnosis of PMR.

The required ACR/EULAR criteria include age over 50, bilateral shoulder aching, and abnormal C-reactive protein or erythrocyte sedimentation rate. Additional criteria are as follows:

1. Morning stiffness >45 min	2 points
2. Hip pain/limited range of motion	1 point
3. Negative rheumatoid factor and anti-citric citrullinated peptide antibodies	2 points
4. Absence of peripheral joint pain (with ultrasonography findings)	1 point
5a. At least one shoulder with subdeltoid bursitis and/or biceps tenosynovitis and/or glenohumeral tenosynovitis (either posterior or axillary) and at least one hip with synovitis and/or trochanteric bursitis	1 point
5b. Both shoulders with subdeltoid bursitis, biceps tendonitis, or glenohumeral synovitis	1 point

A patient with a score of 4 or more (5 if ultrasonography findings are considered) can be categorized as having PMR.

There is no specific laboratory test for PMR; however, laboratory studies that support the diagnosis include positive inflammatory markers C-reactive protein and ESR (the latter must be elevated >40); other findings suggestive for PMR include normochromic normocytic anemia (anemia of chronic disease), thrombocytosis, hypoalbuminemia, and elevated alpha-2 globulin proteins. PMR is distinguished from rheumatoid arthritis by a negative rheumatoid work-up, although in approximately 10% of the elderly population, a nonspecific positive rheumatoid factor is present. Ultrasonography is helpful in visualizing the periarticular inflammatory process including distended, inflamed bursae and tenosynovitis, which helps to differentiate PMR from other rheumatological disease processes.

Goals of care for PMR are to:

- Relieve the chronic pain and inflammation.
- Minimize long-term sequelae or adverse effects of steroid use.
- Maintain optimum physical function.

Treatment of PMR, as for that of GCA, is low-dose glucocorticoids. In fact, some groups have used response to steroid treatment as diagnostic evidence for the disease. Many sufferers obtain significant relief and effective remission; however, the disease is associated with relapses, and corticosteroid therapy may be required for longer periods than would be considered reasonable to prevent outcomes such as osteoporosis, weight gain, and hyperglycemia.

Degenerative Disorders

Advanced age predisposes to frailty, defined as physical weakness related, among other factors such as immune function and nutritional status, to loss of bone mineral density and muscle mass (sarcopenia) often accompanied by osteoarthritis, which combine to result in loss of mobility. Frail elders fall resulting in fractures, myofascial pain, back pain, and other types of injury. Pain itself is implicated in diminished ambulatory capacity, which increases the risk of sustaining an injurious fall with attempted ambulation. The injury then results in pain that reinitiates the vicious cycle of *pain – immobility – fall – injury – pain*. Continued immobility insidiously leads to development of compression fractures, with or without trauma, as well as contractures and pressure ulcers.

Myofascial pain, common in all age groups but especially prevalent in older adults, is effectively and appropriately addressed non-pharmacologically through passive or active range of motion, osteopathic manual medicine techniques, topical heat/cold, appropriate exercise, and other complementary therapies. Weight-bearing exercise is important to prevent osteoporosis as well as for maintenance of muscle strength. The geriatric and physical therapy adages *"if you don't use it you lose it"* and *"motion is lotion"* should motivate clinicians to encourage older individuals to remain as active as possible so as to forestall the development of ambulatory dysfunction and its sequelae.

Osteoarthritis

Arguably the most common cause of pain in persons over age 50, osteoarthritis (OA), also referred to as degenerative joint disease (DJD), is present to some degree in many older persons, with radiographic evidence found in 80% of people over age 75. Most frequently seen in distal fingers, thumbs, neck, lower back, knees, and hips, it is estimated that over 10 million Americans suffer from OA of the knee alone. In the NHANES III study of over 6000 adults over the age of 60, 18.1% men and 23.5% women reported knee pain on most days of preceding 6 weeks. Also seen was a trend for increased knee pain in women and older age. The degree of disability caused by the pain of OA is variable and may be related to the amount of joint destruction, although radiographic findings do not reliably predict the amount of pain an individual may experience.

The pathophysiology of OA is characterized by breakdown and erosion of articular cartilage, either as a primary condition, due to "wear-and-tear" overuse or to direct trauma. OA affects all elements of joints, articular cartilage, bone, and menisci. The injured cartilage becomes soft, frayed, and thinned with sclerosis (eburnation) of subchondral bone and outgrowths of osteophytes at the margins which cause chronic, occasionally severe pain and loss of function.

The strongest determinant of OA is age, with most cases presenting after age 45; it is more common in men under age 45, while most cases after age 45 occur in women, in whom OA of the hand is quite prevalent. Other risk factors for OA are:

- Joint malalignment (e.g., bow-legged or "double-jointed" individuals)
- Weakness of the quadriceps muscles
- Hereditary gene defect affecting cartilage-component collagen
- Joint injury or overuse from physical labor or sports trauma
- Obesity during midlife or later – most strongly predictive

The diagnosis of OA is usually based on history of pain with weight bearing, morning stiffness, and a family history of arthritis. Physical exam reveals hypertrophic osseous structures with crepitance upon passive range of motion, particularly of the knee. Examination may reveal Bouchard's and/or Heberden's nodes, which are bony enlargements in the PIP and DIP joints of the hands. These changes are found more frequently in postmenopausal women and are often associated with a genetic predisposition. Inflammatory changes consisting of tenderness and soft-tissue swelling may occur in the early stages of Heberden's node formation, but this reaction usually subsides in the more chronic stages. The ACR criteria for diagnosis of OA are pain and:

- Age greater than 50 years old
- Morning stiffness lasting less than 30 minutes
- Crepitus
- Bony tenderness
- Bony enlargement
- No palpable warmth
- If at least 3, sensitivity 95%, specificity 69%

While there are no specific laboratory tests for diagnosis of OA, plain radiographs can be very helpful. Characteristic X-ray findings include:

- Osteophyte formation (which correlates with pain)
- Sclerosis
- Joint space narrowing
- Cystic subchondral bone

CT scans and MRIs are usually not necessary; however, standing (weight-bearing) films are useful, and knee radiographs should specifically include weight-bearing anteroposterior and patella sunrise views.

The goals of care for OA are to:

- Minimize symptoms.
- Preserve physical (ambulatory) function.

Nonpharmacologic therapies directed at maintaining function include appropriate exercise, physical therapy, assistive devices, braces, and orthotics. Education about joint preservation and maintenance of physical function is extremely important. Weight loss has shown good evidence of pain reduction and slowed progression of disease. However, some studies find that pain reduction is more correlated with changes in body fat rather than overall weight reduction; thus, exercise to improve overall muscle strength and flexibility (walking, cycling, or swimming) and directed to specific areas (e.g., leg lifts to improve quadriceps strength) is key. Appropriate footwear is also important. Podiatrists may recommend medial or lateral wedge insoles or other orthotics to correct joint alignment. Physical therapy is another important modality for assessing gait and balance, need for assistive devices and for instructing patients in appropriate exercise modalities. Patellar taping, bracing with neoprene sleeves, or unloader brace to decrease medial compartment load may also be helpful.

The American College of Rheumatology lists the following pharmacologic agents for OA:

- Acetaminophen
- NSAIDs
- COX-2 inhibitors
- Analgesics
- Topical agents
- Intra-articular injections

Table 9 is a compilation of pharmaceutical recommendations for treatment of OA from the American College of Rheumatology, the American Geriatrics Society, and the American Pain Society.

Although the above guidelines give no recommendation for their use, topical analgesics that may be helpful include capsaicin cream, lidocaine cream and patch, and NSAID patches, gels, and lotions.

Table 9 Treatment of osteoarthritis

Conditionally recommended	Considerations
Acetaminophen	First choice for mild/moderate pain Starting dose 325–500 mg every 4–6 h Maximum dose 2500 mg/day (not 4000 mg) With renal impairment or hazardous alcohol use/liver disease, cut by 50–75% or consider different therapy Consider around-the-clock administration if pain is continuous
Oral NSAIDs	Several NSAIDs available, COX-2 inhibitors with PPI Widest prescribed class of medications in the world All have demonstrated efficacy for pain Use limited by cardiovascular, GI, and renal toxicity
Topical NSAIDs	Better safety profile than oral NSAIDs, similar efficacy Best if used in patients with one or few joints affected
SNRIs (duloxetine)	Serotonin and norepinephrine reuptake inhibitor May consider in patients who have a contraindication to NSAID use
Tramadol	Mixed opioid and central neurotransmitter mechanism Start low dose, especially in elderly; watch for drowsiness/dizziness; avoid combining with other opioids; use with caution in patients with seizure disorder; titrate dose slowly
Intra-articular injections	Repository corticosteroids Hyaluronate
Do not use	Chondroitin sulfate, glucosamine
Controversial	Opioid analgesics

Adapted from: Hochberg et al. [23], AGS Panel on Persistent Pain in Older Persons [24]
Derry et al. [25]
Wang et al. [26]

The use of opioids for OA pain remains controversial. However, it should be noted that opioid analgesics are, at least from a general medical point of view, a safer option than oral NSAIDs for patients with renal or cardiovascular disease and for those with history of or concern for GI bleeding. Risk factors for developing toxicity from NSAID or COX-2 use are:

- True volume depletion
  - Nausea, vomiting, diarrhea, diuretics, anorexia, poor oral intake
- Effective volume depletion
  - Congestive heart failure, cirrhosis, nephrosis
- Hypertension
  - Treated with BP medications
- Chronic kidney disease
  - Moderate to severe

Clinicians should bear in mind the fact that treatment of osteoarthritis with pharmacologic therapy is palliative; therefore, it must be safe, tolerable, and effective. There is no long-term benefit to most treatments. If the patient does not experience significant symptomatic improvement, there may be no reason for continuing that treatment. Joint replacement surgery is indicated for patients who are unable to obtain adequate analgesia with the above modalities, especially for those whose function is negatively affected.

Spinal Stenosis

Spinal stenosis is an increasingly common cause of persistent radicular pain in the back or legs caused by osteoarthritic changes in the vertebrae that impinge on the central spinal canal causing neuropathic spinal pain. The hallmark presentation of spinal stenosis is the presence of "pseudo-claudication," which is neurogenic pain, i.e., nonvascular in origin, that occurs during ambulation.

Clinical presentation is unusual in patients under the age of 50, and men are twice as likely to be affected as women. Complaints include "heaviness" in the buttocks and/or legs that is aggravated by walking and can progress to severe, searing "claudication" pain. The pain is relieved by rest or by forward bending (as in bending over a shopping cart or walker). Less commonly, lower extremity weakness or atrophy may accompany spinal stenosis.

Diagnosis is based on the classic presentation of pain with ambulation that is relieved or lessened by rest or flexion. There are no specific physical exam findings or provocative maneuvers for diagnosis of spinal stenosis; however, a focused neurologic exam may reveal loss of deep tendon reflexes, pain, and/or vibratory sensation and help pinpoint the level of spinal involvement. Laboratory testing is not needed unless there is concern for infection or malignancy (please see the section on "Low Back Pain – Red Flags." CT scan or MRI can visualize the exact location of foraminal impingement; if neurosurgical intervention is needed, MRI is the neuroimaging procedure of choice.

Goals of care for spinal stenosis are to:

- Assure the patient that the pain is not vascular and/or life-threatening.
- Achieve analgesia sufficient to allow preservation of ambulation.

Treatment options include oral analgesics such as NSAIDs (if tolerated and not contraindicated due to coexisting disease), calcitonin, gabapentin, limaprost, and methylcobalamin. Parenteral, but not intranasal, calcitonin was shown in one study to give transient (less than 3 months) analgesic benefits. Evidence for efficacy of the other medications is limited.

Other options include topical analgesics and interventional procedures such as epidural corticosteroid injections, spinal cord stimulation, and surgical decompression or laminectomy. Physical therapy may assist in identifying ways to improve flexibility, stabilization, and strengthening as well as to identify appropriate assistive devices if needed. Non-weight-bearing exercise, such as aquatherapy, is helpful for maintaining strength and flexibility. Complementary therapy such as acupuncture, application of heat/cold, massage, and joint range of motion or careful spinal manipulation may be helpful. As with all types of persistent pain, a multimodal approach is encouraged.

Compression Fractures

Compression fractures are most commonly caused by loss of bone mineral density due to osteoporosis, but they may also be related to trauma, malignancy (bone metastasis), metabolic disorders, or infection (osteomyelitis). Osteoporosis is defined as diminished bone density 2.5 standard deviations below that of healthy 25-year-old, same sex members of the population. More than 700,000 osteoporotic vertebral compression fractures (VCFs) occur in the USA annually. Predisposing causes of osteoporosis are age, female gender, confinement to bed (non-weight bearing), Caucasian or Asian race, and family history. Secondary causes of osteoporosis include certain disease states, such as malabsorption syndromes, or medications, such as with long-term use of steroids.

VCFs are a source of significant pain and disability in the frail elderly population, especially in older women, and correlate with increased mortality. If severe or multiple, the resulting thoracic kyphosis deformity can lead to diminished lung capacity and respiratory impairment; cardiovascular, musculoskeletal, and immune functions are also adversely affected. In all cases, the discomfort and debility may lead to immobility, isolation, depression, and impaired quality of life.

Patients with vertebral compression fracture may classically present with pain localized to a spinal segment that occurred suddenly while bending or lifting. However, there may be no identifiable precipitating event. Radiographic evidence of thoracic or lumbar compression fractures in asymptomatic patients is not uncommon. The wedge-shaped deformities "wedge fractures" found on X-Ray demonstrate loss of the anterior portion with relative preservation of the posterior height of vertebral bodies. The finding of presence of non-traumatic, non-disease-related VTFs constitutes de facto evidence of osteoporosis.

Diagnosis of compression fractures is made through the history and physical findings of pain localized over vertebral segment(s), loss of axial height, and increased thoracic kyphosis or lumbar lordosis. Plain film radiographs will confirm the diagnosis; CT scans or MRIs are usually not needed unless surgical intervention is contemplated. All patients with VCFs should also undergo evaluation to rule out systemic illness, such as malignancy, infection, and endocrine, renal, or liver disease.

Goals of care for compression fractures are to:

- Stabilize fracture site as necessary.
- Provide analgesia adequate to maintain cardiorespiratory and ambulatory function.
- Prevent further progression of osteoporosis and further fracture.

Healing of VTFs is estimated to take 4 to 6 weeks. Pain management options and interventional techniques for compression fractures include:

- Systemic analgesics
- Intrathecal analgesics

- Corticosteroids
- Physical therapy (gait training, bracing)
- Bracing, interventional techniques (kyphoplasty, vertebroplasty)
- Surgery (vertebral fusion)

Analgesics are needed in the acute phase to allow the patient to maintain mobility and, in the case of thoracic VTF, to maintain respiratory capacity. Adjunctive to pain control, bisphosphonates are drugs that inhibit osteoclastic activity to prevent further loss of bone density; patients who have already fractured are at high risk of incurring another fracture and so should be targeted for therapeutic intervention.

Kyphoplasty or vertebroplasty are recommended for patients with severe, unremitting pain and in those for whom progression of kyphosis or neurologic consequences are likely. Some studies show longer rates of patient survival following vertebral augmentation surgery for VTF, and this may be related to improved physical function, pain control, and overall quality of life.

Contractures and Pressure Ulcers

Arguably the most troublesome outcome of prolonged immobility and/or bed rest is contractures of the extremities and pressure ulcers. While clearly the best treatment for these problems is prevention, in clinical practice, it is not always possible to intervene prior to the development of skin breakdown or contracture.

Contractures are an insidious, progressive problem resulting from neurologic or orthopedic conditions affecting the hands, digits, shoulder, knee, elbow, foot, wrist, hip, and spine. Damaged peripheral or central nervous system function can result from conditions such as spinal cord injury, progressive neurological degeneration (Parkinson disease, dementia), demyelinating syndromes (multiple sclerosis), and following stroke or cerebrovascular injury (hemiparesis or plegia). Extremity contractures also can result from severe burns or congenital nervous system disorders such as cerebral palsy. Contractures also result from fractures and other orthopedic problems. However, in clinical practice, it is most common to see a combination of factors that predispose an individual to the development of contractures.

While contracture pain is the focus of this discussion, the effect of contractures on quality of life, ambulatory ability, and productivity cannot be overlooked. Hand contractures alone (which are among the most commonly occurring contractures in the older adult population) result in significant self-care deficits, impacting such basic activities of daily living as feeding, dressing/grooming, and toileting. Contractures also negatively impact the ability to perform instrumental activities of daily living, such as cooking, dialing a phone, using a computer or TV remote, driving a car, shopping, or enjoying hobbies.

Disuse atrophy is implicated in the development of both upper and lower extremity contractures, once again invoking the geriatric adages ("use it or lose it" and "motion is lotion"). However, once contracture progresses to "tight contracture" (unable to be taken through a normal range of motion with passive stretching), any forced movement of the contracted extremity causes severe pain.

Goals of care for contracture pain include:

- Amelioration of the contracture and prevention of further progression
- Analgesia sufficient to allow range of motion and restorative care

Contracture pain treatment should target attempts at relief of the pain and spasm. An interdisciplinary approach that includes orthopedists, physical therapists, occupational therapists, and nursing and pain management clinicians gives the best chance for reducing both the pain and disability. Oral analgesics, including NSAIDs, tramadol, or other short-acting opioids, should be timed for peak effect during PT/OT sessions or procedures. Spray and stretch techniques using topical anesthetics may be helpful, especially when positioning and splinting the affected extremity(ies). Topical analgesics may be useful for patients too debilitated to take systemic medications, and they have the advantage of being placed directly at the site of contracture pain. Osteopathic or other manual medicine techniques to assist with joint mobilization and normalization of range of motion are important therapeutic adjuncts. Complementary and alternative medicine techniques including balneotherapy, massage, and behavioral therapy should also be integrated into the plan of care to help achieve better quality of life and function.

Pressure ulcers, likewise, often result from loss of normal nervous system function; fully sensate individuals will reposition themselves (or at least squirm around) when an area of pressure begins to develop pain. Pressure ulcers result during prolonged bedrest in terminally ill patients, in acute medical conditions and/or sedation such as needed in the setting of an ICU, or during prolonged anesthesia for surgery. In the geriatric population, pressure ulcers occur in those who are rendered bedbound due to severe dementia, debility, deconditioning, and frailty.

While studies suggest that 50% of patients with pressure ulcers report pain, this number is complicated by both the complexity of the type of pain experienced at the site of a pressure ulcer (at rest, during repositioning, during dressing changes or other procedures) and the fact that many individuals with pressure ulcers are unable to self-report due to advanced disease states or dementia. From the perspective of palliative care, analgesics should be provided to cover both baseline (at rest) pain and incident (during treatment or activity) pain. Patients who are able should be asked to rate their pain using a pain scale appropriate to the patient's situation, i.e., self-report versus caregiver observation. Medication titration may be directed by response to treatment as measured on the scale.

Some patients with pressure ulcers report that "keeping still" relieves their pain and that pressure-relieving or wound care equipment (wound VACs) are significant inciting sources of pain. In any case, "keeping still" is how the problem originated and is therefore not a good plan of care option.

Goals of care for pressure ulcer pain include:

- Baseline, around-the-clock analgesia sufficient to allow comfort during repositioning and to encourage movement
- Preemptive pain medications administered prior to dressing changes or other procedures, such as personal care and toileting

Systemic, around-the-clock analgesics, as indicated for mild to moderate pain, are the standard of care for pressure ulcer pain. Topical modalities are problematic due to the presence of the wound itself, and interventional procedures are usually reserved for patients who will require surgery. Surgical debridement of necrotic pressure ulcers is extremely painful, however, and warrants strong analgesics such as oral or IV opioids. As noted above, an interdisciplinary, multimodal approach to the care of frail older patients is always the best treatment option.

It bears repeating that, in the case of pain from contractures or pressure ulcers, "an ounce of prevention is worth a pound of cure."

Low Back Pain

Chronic low back pain (LBP), defined as pain that persists for greater than 12 weeks, is one of the leading reasons patients seek medical care. Common causes include muscle strain/sprain, arthritis, sciatica, spinal stenosis, or herniated disk, but in older adults, there may be a more serious cause underlying a complaint of LBP. Fortunately, there are many available guidelines to assist clinicians in evaluating a new complaint of LBP.

The 2007 Joint Clinical Practice Guideline from the American College of Physicians (ACP) and the American Pain Society (APS) gives strong recommendation, based on moderate-quality evidence, to perform a focused history and physical with the goal of placing LBP sufferers into one of three categories:

1. Nonspecific LBP
2. Pain potentially associated with radiculopathy or spinal stenosis
3. Back pain associated with another spinal cause for which prompt treatment is necessary or a specific treatment exists

Focused history and physical should seek the location, duration, and frequency of the LBP and whether it represents new onset or a flare of a previous pain. Some questions to consider are:

- Does the pain respond to rest or is it improved by light exercise?
- Does the pain radiate to the hip, groin, or flank?
- Does the pain awaken the patient from sleep?
- Does the patient have a history of cancer, IV drug or chronic steroid use, or trauma?

The history should include an assessment of psychologic risk factors which may predict an individual's risk for developing chronic, disabling back pain.

The search for a cause of LBP is complicated by the anatomic fact that multiple abdominal structures relate to a relatively small area on the sensory homunculus, making exact localization of pain difficult. Pinprick discrimination is much less precise than on other areas of the body such as the face or hands. It may therefore be difficult to determine whether the source of pain is visceral, arthrodial, or myotomal. For example, visceral pain can mimic myofascial pain, such as in the case of LBP referred from an abdominal area aneurysm.

An evaluation of the pattern of the LBP should seek signs of radicular distribution, neurologic changes (especially of the lower extremities and/or bowel or bladder incontinence), or non-spinal (e.g., referred) sources of pain. Deep tendon reflexes, pinprick sensation, Patrick's (FABER) test, and heel and toe walk evaluate for neurologic involvement.

"Red flags" or "yellow flags" are findings in a patient with LBP that may point to non-musculoskeletal causes. Red flags should alert clinicians that the etiology of the LBP may be more serious, while yellow flags herald a more benign cause.

Red flag concerns include:

- Malignancy
  - Non-skin cancer
  - Age over 50
  - Unexplained weight loss
  - No relief with rest
  - Elevated ESR
  - Spinal tenderness
- Spinal infection
  - History of immunodeficiency
  - History of IV drug abuse
  - History of skin or urinary tract infection
- Cauda equina syndrome
  - Urinary retention
  - Bilateral lower extremity weakness
  - "Saddle" anesthesia

Yellow flag factors include:

- Psychological factors
  - Current life stressors
  - Fear-avoidance behaviors[a]
  - Coping skills
  - Somatization[a]
  - History of abuse/trauma
  - Depression[a]/anxiety
  - Personality disorders
- Pain factors
  - Severity of symptoms[a]
  - Impaired function
- Social factors
  - Job dissatisfaction[a]
  - Disputed workman's compensation claims[a]
  - Work characteristics
  - Secondary gain

[a]May predict potential for long-term disability

LBP that awakens the patient at night is concerning for a cause related to a structure outside the back, and LBP that is constant and fails to respond to usual care or improve with time must prompt further work-up. With respect to red flag findings, the presence of fever or recent skin or urinary tract infection should raise concern for an infectious etiology for the LBP, while history of weight loss, fatigue, or anorexia may point to malignancy as causative, especially in those with a history of cancer. Sudden onset of bowel and bladder dysfunction is an ominous finding that requires immediate evaluation for spinal cord compression. Any of these findings should prompt immediate imaging with MRI or CT scans and referral to appropriate specialists.

The Agency for Health Care Policy and Research (AHCPR) lists the following criteria as giving more weight to a specific, non-musculoskeletal cause for LBP:

Recent significant trauma or milder trauma in those aged <50	Fracture
Osteoporosis	Fracture
Unexplained weight loss	Cancer
Immunosuppressive therapy	Cancer
Unexplained fever or recent urinary tract infection	Infection
Intravenous drug use	Infection
Prolonged use of glucocorticoids	Fracture, infection
Age greater than 70	Fracture, cancer
Pain lasting longer than 6 weeks	Cancer, infection
History of cancer	Cancer
Progressive motor or sensory deficit	Cauda equina syndrome
Saddle anesthesia, bowel/bladder incontinence or retention	Cauda equina syndrome

Having ruled out one of the above etiologies, the most common cause of LBP that remains is musculoskeletal or somatic dysfunction, which implies that the pain is not due to underlying serious pathology. This type of LBP may be designated as strain/sprain, mechanical or "idiopathic" LBP. Mechanical LBP due to muscle strain or sprain can have associated radicular symptoms, such as sciatica (radiation of the pain down the posterior aspect of an affected leg and into the foot). Radicular pain may herald the presence of a herniated nucleus pulposus or disk. Most cases of mechanical LBP, with or without herniated disk or disk disease/degeneration, will resolve within 6 weeks to 6 months.

Another common cause of LBP in all age groups, especially seen in women of tall stature, is piriformis syndrome, diagnosed by characteristic pain in the buttock lateral to the spine. When asked to point to the cause of pain, the patient may indicate a point midway between the iliac crest and base of the spine where the examiner can palpate an olive-shaped mass: spasm of the piriformis muscle. Piriformis syndrome is triggered by sitting too long in one position. In addition to postural adaptation to avoid its development, analgesics and specific osteopathic manipulative techniques are helpful to relieve piriformis spasm and pain. Piriformis muscle injections with or without botulinum toxin can benefit as well.

Additional discussion of other types of persistent back pain in older adults can be found within this chapter's sections on spinal stenosis, osteoarthritis, and compression fractures.

The goals of care for persistent LBP are to:

- Achieve analgesia sufficient to allow optimum physical function
- Maintain or restore ambulatory capacity
- Prevent progression or recurrence of the pain

Treatment options for LBP rely on an understanding of the etiology of the pain. Treatment of mechanical LBP should be directed at early mobilization and maintenance of ambulatory function. This is best accomplished with multimodal therapy including physical therapy, osteopathic or other forms of manual medicine, appropriate exercise prescription, and analgesics as needed. Skeletal muscle relaxants may be helpful to relieve spasm in the acute phase of strain/sprain LBP or piriformis syndrome; however, the use of these agents for more than a few days is discouraged even in younger persons. They are usually contraindicated in frail older adults due to the risk of their causing cognitive dysfunction, sedation, confusion, and falls.

As noted, for a more thorough review of analgesic options for other causes of LBP (compression fracture, spinal stenosis, or bony metastasis), please refer to those sections within this chapter. The prognosis for resolution of LBP depends on the cause of the problem. Mechanical LBP and pain from disk herniation are usually amenable to conservative therapy based on the goals of early ambulation and return to function. For those who fail to respond to usual care, referral for orthopedic and/or neurosurgical evaluation may be indicated.

Central Pain Processing Disorders

Scientific understanding of pain physiology has advanced considerably in the last several decades. It is known that, under certain conditions, nociceptive peripheral afferents can trigger prolonged increase in the excitability of central nervous system neurons, resulting in an amplified or augmented pain response. Persistent nociceptive input (inflammation, injury, neural irritation) results in neuroplasticity which induces changes in both the peripheral and central nervous systems such that painful sensations arise independent of noxious stimuli. This nociceptive dysregulation has been referred to as "central sensitization."

The clinical consequence of central sensitization is that affected individuals experience pain that is amplified in excess of the stimulus that produced it, such as seen in allodynia, hyperesthesia, phantom pain, or expansion/persistence of the painful field around an initial injury. Certain pain diagnoses have the characteristic finding of central sensitization in common: fibromyalgia, poststroke pain, postoperative pain such as anterior chest wall syndromes seen in mastectomy or thoracotomy patients, post-amputation phantom limb pain, as well as some types of chronic low back pain. Recognition and basic understanding of central sensitization and its relationship to abnormal pain processing are helpful in aiding the clinical approach to patients who present with these types of pain.

Fibromyalgia

Fibromyalgia (FM) may be regarded as a prototype painful condition due to central sensitization. FM affects only 2–7% of the population, but the disability associated with FM is significant. Diffuse widespread tenderness, characterized by spontaneous pain above and below the diaphragm on both sides of the body with no other apparent cause, defines the presentation of FM. Sufferers also have comorbid diagnoses of migraine, irritable bowel syndrome (IBS), other neuropathies, and mood or cognitive disorders and/or anxiety.

FM occurs with a ratio of 9:1 women to men. It usually presents in the second or third decade but may take up to 5 years to diagnose. Although most clinicians eschew the "tender point" exam, FM has been defined as the presence of 11 out of 18 tender points. In 2010, the American College of Rheumatology (ACR) revised the guidelines for diagnosing FM to focus on the findings of widespread pain at multiple sites on both sides and in three out of four quadrants of the body.

Patients with FM present with multiple symptomatic complaints in addition to pain. They may experience generalized stiffness, cognitive effects ("fibro fog"), bowel and bladder complaints (IBS, interstitial cystitis), weakness, or fatigue and sleep disturbances. A patient satisfies the 2010 ACR guidelines diagnostic criteria for fibromyalgia if the following three conditions are met:

- Widespread pain index (WPI) ≥ 7 and symptom severity (SS) scale score ≥ 5 or WPI 3–6 and SS scale score ≥ 9.
- Symptoms have been present at a similar level for at least 3 months.
- The patient does not have a disorder that would otherwise explain the pain.

Goals of care for fibromyalgia are to:

- Acknowledge to the patient that the pain is real.
- Seek combination of therapies to achieve analgesia and quality of life.
- Provide supportive care and encouragement for maintained physical activity and overall psychosocial function.

Historically, patients with FM have received "usual treatment" for some or all of the above symptoms, such as NSAIDs, acetaminophen, or opioids for the pain/tenderness, skeletal muscle relaxants for the stiffness, antidepressants and/or anxiolytics, and sedative-hypnotics for sleep. This piecemeal approach should be avoided as none of these medications have been shown to be of value. Current knowledge points toward treating FM as a central processing disorder with SNRIs (duloxetine, milnacipran) or alpha-2 delta ligand, pregabalin.

Table 10 shows the current pharmacotherapy for FM.

There is currently no cure for FM, and patients have shown best results with multimodal therapy that incorporates pharmacologic and nonpharmacologic approaches. There is good evidence that FM symptoms benefit from appropriate aerobic exercise, taking care not to "overdo" it and cause a flare or excessive fatigue,

Table 10 Current pharmacotherapy for FM

FDA approved	APS, EULAR guidelines – additional agents
Duloxetine	TCAs (amitriptyline, desipramine)
	Cyclobenzaprine
Milnacipran	SSRIs (fluoxetine)
Pregabalin	Tramadol, gabapentin
	Sleep, antianxiety medications (trazodone, benzodiazepines, nonbenzodiazepine sedatives, L-dopa, and carbidopa)
	Pramipexole

Burckhardt et al. [27], Carville et al. [28], Uceyler et al. [29], Lunn et al. [30] and Tzellos et al. [31]

and cognitive behavioral therapy has been shown to help with the cognitive and mood disorders as well as for improving sleep and overall quality of life.

Persistent Postsurgical Pain

Older individuals undergo surgeries of every type, both elective and emergent. Clearly, older age correlates with higher risk for operative complications, not least among them intractable or persistent pain. Examples of persistent postsurgical pain (PPSP) include post-thoracotomy pain, anterior chest wall syndrome, postmastectomy pain, and phantom limb pain following amputation. A 2005 survey indicated that 62% of geriatric patients experienced acute severe postsurgical pain although 87% reported satisfaction with the treatment received for their pain. In order to prevent PSP, acute post-op pain must be well-managed.

Central sensitization can develop from all types of inadequately treated pain, so that the perioperative period is critical for identifying patients at risk and for implementing steps to prevent both acute and persistent postsurgical pain. Safe, effective intraoperative anesthesia and postoperative analgesia are the goal.

The leading operative complication in older adults is myocardial infarction; other complications range from sepsis to deep venous thrombosis, pulmonary emboli, and death. Another operative consequence that is less recognized yet of equal concern is the neurotoxicity that results from anesthetic metabolites: aging brains are more vulnerable to drug effects that can precipitate mental status changes. Post-op confusion as a side effect of anesthesia is common but usually short-lived. A far more dangerous (and potentially life-threatening) mental status change in older surgical patients is delirium, especially in patients with impaired renal function.

A postanesthesia, mild cognitive decline or transient confusional state may be subtle and characterized by changes in one or more neuropsychologic domains, whereas postoperative delirium is defined as an acute confusional state with alterations in attention and consciousness. Pre-existing comorbidities, other factors such as medications, and post-op complications are contributory, but a leading avoidable cause of delirium is adverse drug reactions. Several studies support a role for meperidine in causing increased risk of delirium in elderly surgical patients. It is important for all clinicians to carefully assess patients preoperatively for factors such as chronic kidney disease or dehydration that may adversely affect the use of pre- and intraoperative anesthetic agents as well as post-op analgesics.

Goals of care for acute postsurgical pain are to:

- Prevent central sensitization and PPSP through adequate operative analgesia.
- Provide analgesia sufficient to allow optimum recovery and to facilitate early ambulation and return to normal function.
- Prevent adverse events due to drug accumulation.
- Identify and address consequences of postsurgical pain such as immobility (pressure ulcers, contractures) or mental status changes (delirium).

Assiduous evaluation for risk and potentially causative factors coupled with cautious use of medications are the best defense against adverse postsurgical outcomes, including PPSP, diminished functional capacity, and mental status decline. Consideration of age-related physiologic changes must inform the choice of analgesic(s), dosages, and routes of administration for older surgical candidates: specifically, hepatic function (metabolism) and renal function (excretion).

In short, treatment of acute surgical pain is needed to avoid the potential for development of PPSP – yet it must not be at the expense of a safe, uncomplicated recovery. A concise review of key physiologic concerns includes:

- Hepatic function changes.
  - For example, cytochrome P450 system declines in efficiency with age
    - No single easy test to evaluate the liver for ability to metabolize drugs
    - Best indices of impaired hepatic metabolic capacity are:
      - Low albumin concentration, elevated INR or prothrombin ratio
      - More predictable in chronic liver dysfunction
      - May be seen in acute liver dysfunction
      - May be influenced by other factors, e.g., poor nutritional state
- Renal function progressively declines with age.
  - For example, meperidine should be avoided since excretion of the toxic metabolite normeperidine is often delayed, causing direct toxicity
    - Caution in use of drugs that affect renal function
    - Dose adjustment needed for renally excreted analgesics
    - Creatinine clearance rather than serum Cr should be used for making dose adjustments.

Many analgesic medications have renal effects, including NSAIDs and opioids. NSAIDs have potential for direct renal toxicity and should be completely avoided or used with caution, especially in older patients with comorbid conditions such as congestive heart failure, diabetes, or volume depletion.

With respect to opioids, the kidney accounts for about 90% of the excretion of opioid parent drug and metabolites. Reduced excretion of most opioids leads to accumulation of active or toxic metabolites which may result in increased analgesia, sedation, and respiratory depression. Since the "gold standard" for analgesia is morphine, a review of its metabolism and elimination may assist clinicians in determining which patients may benefit and which may be harmed. Morphine is metabolized in the liver to form the following metabolites:

- Morphine-3-glucuronide (M-3-G)
- Morphine-6-glucuronide (M-6-G)
- Morphine-3-6-diglucuronide normorphine and 3-ethereal sulfate (in lesser amounts)

Due to substantial extrahepatic morphine conjugation, in patients with mild hepatic insufficiency, morphine metabolism is not significantly affected; however, in patients with severe hepatic dysfunction, morphine has a prolonged elimination half-life which can result in the adverse effect of increased sedation.

M-3-G is inactive at opioid receptors, while M-6-G is twice as potent an analgesic as morphine. Accumulation of morphine metabolites in renal failure, particularly M-6-G, will lead to morphine intoxication which is manifested by prolonged central nervous system and respiratory depression and/or neurologic side effects such as myoclonus. A good rule of thumb when determining morphine dosage for patients with impaired renal function is to reduce the dose by:

- 75% for GFR less than 10 mL/min
- 50% for GFR between 10 and 20 mL/min
- 25% for GFR between 20 and 50 mL/min

Hydromorphone is a morphine analogue with shorter duration of action and similar pharmacokinetics and pharmacodynamics. It is a hydrophilic opioid with strong mu receptor affinity. Its metabolite, hydromorphone-3-glucuronide, appears to be pharmacologically inactive. Although reduced liver function results in higher plasma concentration (due to decreased first pass metabolism), there is no significant effect on plasma elimination. Therefore, with careful dosing and titration, hydromorphone is a better analgesic choice for patients with renal insufficiency or failure.

Table 11 is an overview of available short-acting opioids and suggested starting doses for use in postsurgical pain

For frail elderly surgical patients, APS guidelines recommend reducing the opioid dose by up to 50% and titrating upward based on therapeutic response. If it is deemed necessary to initiate therapy at a lower dose, start with oxymorphone 5 mg (or equianalgesic equivalent of another opioid) and titrate to pain response.

Table 12 lists long-acting opioids to be used once a baseline dose has been established in an opioid-tolerant patient. Opioid tolerance is defined as 60 mg of morphine daily (or its equianalgesic equivalent) for 1 week or more.

Table 11 Opioid options for postsurgical pain

Drug	PO (mg)	IV/IM (mg)	Timing (h)
Codeine	30–60	120	3–4
Hydrocodone	5–10	NA	3–4
Hydromorphone	7.5	0.2–0.4	3–4 (5–10 min for IV/IM)
Morphine	15–30	5–10	3–4 (5–20 min for IV/IM)
Oxycodone	10–30	NA	3–4
Oxymorphone	10–20	NA	4–6
Tramadol	50–100	NA	6
Fentanyl	NA	25–50 ug	5–10 min

Table 12 Long-acting opioids for postsurgical pain (opioid-tolerant patient)

Morphine	Frequency	Starting dose	Comments
Avinza	q 24 h	30 mg q 24 h; adjust increments <30 mg q 4 d	60, 90, 120 mg only in opioid-tolerant pts
Kadian	q 12 or 24	No systematic evaluation	Initially only 20 mg, incr. no >than 20 mg q 48 h
MS Contin	q 12	No systematic evaluation	200 mg dose only in opioid-tolerant pts
Oramorph	q 12	No systematic evaluation	
Oxycodone			
OxyContin	q 12	10 mg q 12; total daily dose incr. by 25–50% at ea. Incr.	80 and 160 mg only in opioid-tolerant pts.
Oxymorphone			
Opana ER	q 12	5 mg q 12; individual dosing titration recommended	Titrate at increments of 5–10 mg q 12 h q 3–7d
Fentanyl			
Duragesic	q 72	25 mcgm patch	Only in opioid-tolerant pts

There has been significant inquiry into whether the mode of analgesia delivery may affect surgical outcomes. Some considerations regarding anesthetic and analgesic administration options include:

- Intrathecal/epidural morphine has the theoretical advantage of delivery of opioids in close proximity to spinal cord opioid receptors.
- Intravenous morphine with or without patient-controlled analgesic (PCA) pump improves analgesia.
- Preemptive analgesia initiated before and during surgery in order to reduce consequences of nociceptive transmission may be "protective".
- Anti-hyperalgesic drugs may interfere with induction and maintenance of sensitization:
  – NMDA receptor antagonists (ketamine, dextromethorphan)
  – Gabapentin
  – NSAIDs, COX-2

A systematic review by Fong [11] showed that despite significantly less pain in patients with epidural administration of anesthetics, there was no concurrent reduction in rates of delirium. The effect of preemptive analgesia, while compelling in terms of the theoretical advantage of preventing central sensitization, has shown variable and conflicting results in large studies.

A painful consequence of opioid therapy is the development of postoperative ileus. Since opioid receptors are present throughout the body, including the GI tract, laxatives should be instituted at the time of surgery and during the entire course of treatment with opioid analgesics. Opioid binding at gut receptors can cause bloating, nausea/vomiting, and constipation or ileus. Traditional preventive therapy includes a stool softener (docusate sodium) coupled with a mucosal irritant laxative (sennosides); however, bisacodyl, lactulose, or sorbitol may also be used. Enemas are invasive and uncomfortable and should be reserved for patients who fail to respond to usual therapy.

For intractable constipation or post-op ileus due to opioid use, the peripherally acting mu opioid receptor antagonist methylnaltrexone may be administered. Methylnaltrexone is designed to block the adverse effects of opioid analgesics on the GI tract without blocking their beneficial analgesic effects; it is administered subcutaneously and is very effective in producing laxation.

Relief of pain from surgical procedures is a crucial objective for preventing the development of postoperative persistent pain syndromes. Here again, an ounce of prevention is worth a pound of cure. Clinicians caring for geriatric patients must seek a balance between effective, consistent analgesia and side effects or frank adverse events from the use of analgesics.

Finally, for patients who develop PPSP, goals of care should be directed at the cause of the pain. Phantom limb pain, anterior chest wall pain, and many other forms of PPSP are centrally mediated or "central pain syndromes" and will respond to analgesics typically used for neuropathic pain. A review of medications that are approved for this use may be found in the section on painful diabetic peripheral neuropathy and Table 4.

Intractable forms of PPSP may require adjunctive modalities such as TENS units and nerve blocks. Complementary and alternative therapies should be sought as part of a multimodal plan of care for PPSP.

Central Poststroke Pain

Lesions of the central nervous system can result in pain syndromes which are referred to as central pain. This type of pain, since it results from damage of neuronal tissue, is considered to be neuropathic pain. Causes of central pain include trauma, vascular, infectious, inflammatory, demyelinating, hereditary, and neoplastic conditions; however, the most common cause of central pain resulting from brain injury is that resulting from stroke or central poststroke pain (CPC).

CPC may result from lesions occurring at any level from the foramen magnum to the cerebral cortex. Paradoxically, it is not uncommon for patients with central pain following a brain lesion to exhibit no clearly detectable sensory loss. Once thought to occur only as the result of thalamic lesions, it is now known that this type of central pain can occur from any brain lesion that impacts sensory processing areas.

Important general characteristics of central pain such as central poststroke pain (CSP) include the following:

- Central pain results from injury to somatosensory pathways in the central nervous system (spinal cord or brain).
- The injury may be massive or minimal; some individuals with central pain have no obvious sensory loss despite the severe pain.
- The onset of pain following the injury may be delayed.
- The pain is sometimes reversible.
- Three main components of central pain are:
  - Pain evoked by stimulation
  - Steady and neuralgic-like pain
  - Spontaneous pain
- The pathophysiology of central pain is not well understood.
- Treating central pain successfully can be very challenging.

The onset of CSP may be immediate, commonly occurring during the first year following stroke. Less commonly, CSP may have onset more than 1 year after the injury. Interestingly, types of brain central pain have also been reported to be reversed following a stroke or following the removal of a brain tumor. Of equal interest and contrary to what would be expected, traumatic brain injury and craniotomy sometimes do not result in central pain.

Loss of motor control of various muscle groups (hemiplegia) as a consequence of stroke can itself be quite painful. Motor loss may be focal, multifocal, or generalized. If not addressed and properly treated, it can lead to contractures with resultant increased disability, as covered in a previous section.

Neuroimaging studies including MRI and in certain instances CT/myelography are useful diagnostic modalities when evaluating and treating a patient with CSP.

Goals of care for CSP are to:

- Provide analgesia sufficient to enable therapy that preserves and improves function.
- Achieve quality of life in face of sensory and motor loss.

Unfortunately, strategies to prevent CSP once the cerebrovascular accident has occurred are unknown. The nonpharmacologic approach to a poststroke patient should be directed toward evaluation and treatment of associated neurological impairment, which may include pulmonary care/respiratory therapy, urologic care, wound care, optimizing wheelchair/general seating and positioning, treatment of spasticity and potentially painful muscle spasms, and proper nutrition. Early intervention should involve an interdisciplinary approach that includes physical and occupational therapy.

Management of CSP is complicated by the fact that although many treatments have been attempted, few have been consistently helpful. The FDA has approved pregabalin for the treatment of spinal cord injury pain, and gabapentin, which has a similar mechanism of action as pregabalin, may be helpful. Other medications that may provide some benefit to patients with CSP include:

- Amitriptyline
- Desipramine
- Carbamazepine
- Lamotrigine
- Nonsteroidal anti-inflammatory agents
- Clonazepam
- Oral baclofen
- Tizanidine

Both baclofen and tizanidine are used to control spasticity but also may have analgesic qualities as well. Medications that have not been shown to be helpful for spinal cord-related central pain include trazodone, valproic acid, and mexiletine. The above medications may be considered for brain injury-related central pain, and some studies have suggested that naloxone or propofol may be helpful as well. The use of opioid analgesics for treating the chronic pain associated with spinal cord-related central pain and CSP has shown inconsistent results.

Interventional therapies for CSP have been utilized but again with mixed and often disappointing results. Peripheral nerve blocks may offer temporary but not sustained pain relief. Intravenous lidocaine infusions may result in temporary pain relief, and some patients have experienced prolonged benefit with repeated infusions; however, these should be administered only in a monitored environment supervised by an experienced practitioner.

The use of botulinum toxin injection should be considered when painful spasticity and/or painful muscle spasms associated with CSP are present. For some patients with more generalized spasticity, the use of intrathecal baclofen via an implanted pump may be more appropriate than the use of botulinum toxin injections. Many patients with severe and widespread painful spasticity due to brain or spinal cord injury may actually benefit from both of these modalities. In this instance, the use of intraspinal baclofen would be helpful in reducing the more generalized spasticity, and the use of botulinum toxin would be targeted in a more localized manner to address those areas that may be more resistant to treatment with intrathecal baclofen. These treatments combined or used singly certainly need to be individualized in a patient-centered manner to address the patient-specific needs. Other intraspinal treatment approaches for central pain include the use of intraspinal morphine, clonidine, or ziconotide.

The above treatments are highly specialized and should only be offered by those practitioners with sufficient training and experience to do so. Particularly with respect to the use of intraspinal therapies, monitoring and ongoing care is not only vital to the success of the treatment but is necessary and imperative from a patient safety perspective. In order for these modalities to be used properly, it must be clear that the patient can and will be followed as closely as required by a properly trained and experienced practitioner for all aspects of intraspinal pump/medication management, including but not restricted to dose adjustment, pump refills, and all aspects of pump troubleshooting.

Neurosurgical procedures such as deep brain stimulation or motor cortex stimulation, while generally not helpful for patients with spinal cord injury-related central pain, have been used with varying degrees of success (0–80%) for patients with central poststroke pain.

As with all types of persistent pain, older adults with CSP will benefit from a multimodal, interdisciplinary approach with emphasis on maintenance of function and preservation of quality of life.

References

1. American Geriatrics Society Updated Beers Criteria for Potentially Inappropriate Mediciation Use in Older Adults. The American Geriatrics Society. Beer's criteria update expert panel. J Am Geriatr Soc. 2012;2012:1–16.
2. American Geriatrics Society Panel on the Pharmacological Management of Persistent Pain in Older Persons. Pharmacological management of persistent pain in older persons. J Am Geriatr Soc. 2009;57(8):1331–46.
3. Hanlon JT, Backonja M, Weiner D, Argoff C. Evolving pharmacologic management of persistent pain in older persons. Pain Med. 2009;10(6):959–61.
4. Herr K. Pain assessment strategies in older patients. J Pain. 2011;3(S–1):S-3–13.
5. Bennett MI, Rayment C, Hjermstad M, Aass N, Caraceni A, Stein K. Prevalence and aetiology of pain in cancer patients: a systematic review. Pain. 2012;153:359–65.
6. Paice JA, Ferrell B. The management of cancer pain. CA Cancer J Clin. 2011;61(3):157–82.
7. Barrett AM, Lucero MA, Le T, Robinson RL, Dworkin RH, Chappell AS. Epidemiology, public health burden, and treatment of diabetic peripheral neuropathic pain: a review. Pain Med. 2007;8(S2):S50–62.
8. Galer BS, et al. Assessment of pain quality in chronic neuropathic and nociceptive pain clinical trials with the neuropathic pain scale. J Pain. 2005;6(2):98–106.
9. Backonja M, et al. Painful diabetic neuropathy: epidemiology, natural history, early diagnosis, and treatment options. Pain Med. 2008;9(6):660–74.
10. Bouhassira D, et al. Neuropathic pain phenotyping as a predictor of treatment response in painful diabetic neuropathy:data from the randomized, double-blind, COMB-DN Study. Pain. 2014;155(10):2171–9.
11. Fong H, et al. The role of posterative analgesia in delirium and cognitive decline in elderly patients: a systematic review. Anesth Analg. 2006;102:1225–66.
12. Kroenke K, et al. Gen Hosp Psychiatry. 2009;31(3):206–19.
13. Galvagno, et al. Resid Staff Physician. 2007;53(4)
14. Argoff C, Silvershein D. Mayo Clin Proc. 2009;84(7):602–12.
15. Rowbotham M, et al. Gabapentin for the treatment of postherpetic neuralgia: a randomized controlled trial. JAMA. 1998;280:1837–42.
16. Dworkin RH, et al. Pregabalin for the treatment of postherpetic neuralgia: a randomized, placebo-controlled trial. Neurology. 2003;60:1274–83.
17. Pappagallo M, Haldey EJ. CNS Drugs. 2003;17:771–80.
18. Watson CPN, Babul N. Efficacy of oxycodone in neuropathic pain: a randomized trial in postherpetic neuralgia. Neurology. 1998;50:1837–41.
19. Raja SN, et al. Opioids versus antidepressants in postherpetic neuralgia: a randomized, placebo-controlled trial. Neurology. 2002;59:1015–21.
20. Davies PS, Galer BS. Review of lidocaine patch 5% studies in the treatment of postherpetic neuralgia. Drugs. 2004;64:937–47.
21. Watson CPN, et al. A randomized, vehicle-controlled study of topical capsaicin in postherpetic neuralgia. Clin Ther. 1993;15:510–26.

22. Derry S, et al. Cochrane Database Syst Rev. 2013
23. Hochberg MC, et al. American College of Rheumatology 2012 Recommendations for the use of nonpharmacologic and pharmacologic therapies in osteoarthritis of the hand, hip and knee. Arthritis Care Res. 2012;64(4):465–74.
24. AGS Panel on Persistent Pain in Older Persons. The Management of Persistent Pain in Older Patients. JAGS. 2002;6:S205–24. 2000 Update Arthritis & Rheumatism. 2000;9;1905–15. Guideline for the Management of Pain in OA, RA, and Juvenile Chronic Arthritis. American Pain Society. Second Edition 2002.
25. Derry S, Moore RA, Rabbie R. Topical NSAIDS for chronic musculoskeletal pain in adults. Cochrane Database Syst Rev. 2012;(9):CD007400.
26. Wang ZY, Shi SY, Li SJ, et al. Efficacy and safety of duloxetine on osteoarthritis knee pain: a meta-analysis of randomized controlled trials. Pain Med. 2015;16:1373.
27. Burckhardt C, et al. Guideline for the management of fibromyalgia syndrome pain in adults and children. American Pain Society: Glenview; 2005.
28. Carville SF, et al. Ann Rheum Dis. 2008;67:536–41.
29. Uceyler N, Sommer C, Walitt B, Hauser W. Anticonvulsants for fibromyalgia. Cochrane Database Syst Rev. 2013;(10):CD010782.
30. Lunn MP, et al. Duloxetine for treating painful neuropathy, chronic pain or fibromyalgia. Cochrane Database Syst Rev. 2014;(1):CD007115.
31. Tzellos TG, et al. Gabapentin and pregabalin in the treatment of fibromyalgia: a systematic review and meta-analysis. J Clin Pharm Ther. 2010;35:639.

Further Reading

American Pain Society Guideline for the Management of Cancer Pain in Adults and Children. Clinical Practice Guideline No. 3. Glenview IL; American Pain Society 2005.
Chou R, et al. Opioid treatment guidelines: clinical guidelines for the use of chronic opioid therapy in chronic noncancer pain. J Pain. 2009;10(2):113–30.
James SF, Chahine EB, Sucher AJ, Hanna C. Shingrix: the new adjuvanted recombinant herpes zoster vaccine. Ann Pharmacother. 2018;52(7):673–80.
Gagliese L. Pain and aging: the emergence of a new subfield of pain research. J Pain. 2009;10(4):343–53.
Hadjistavropoulos T, Herr K, Turk DC, et al. An interdisciplinary consensus statement on assessment of pain in older persons. Clin J Pain. 2007;23(Suppl 1):S1–S43.
Herr K. Pain assessment strategies in older patients. J Pain. 2011;3(S–1):S-3–13.
Higginson IS, Murtagh F. Cancer pain epidemiology. In: Bruera ED, Portenoy RK, editors. Cancer pain. 2nd ed. New York: Cambridge University Press; 2010. p. 37–52.
McAuliffe L, Nay R, O-Donnell M, Fetherstonhaugh D. Pain assessment in older people with dementia: literature review. J Adv Nursing. 2009;65(1):2–10.
Partidge JSL, Harari D, Martin FC, Dhesi JK. The impact of pre-operative comprehensive geriatric assessment on postoperative outcomes in older patients undergoingscheduled surgery: a systematic review. Anaesthesia. 2014;69(Suppl. 1):8–16.
Pipitone N, Salvarini C. Update on polymyalgia rheumatica. Eur J Intern Med. 2013;24(7):583–9.
Razq M, Balicas M, Mankan N. Use of hydromorphone and morphine for patients with hepatic and renal impairment. Am J Therap. 2007;14:414–6.
Reiser L. Pharmacological management of persistent pain in older persons. J Pain. 2011;12(3 S–1):S21–9.
Sauaia A, Min S, et al. Postoperative pain management in elderly patients: correlation between adherence to treatment guidelines and patient satisfaction. JAGS. 2005;53:274–82.
Woolf CJ. Central sensitization: implications for the diagnosis and treatment of pain. Pain. 2011;152:S5–S15.

Recommendations for Classes of Medications in Older Adults

Adam J. Carinci, Scott Pritzlaff, and Alex Moore

Introduction

While chronic pain is one of the most prevalent conditions found in elderly patients, few studies investigating the effects of analgesic drugs have been performed specifically in older people. In a recent literature review, eight studies were found which evaluated the prevalence of "current" pain in older people. This review found that 20–46% of older people living in the general community and 28–73% of those living in residential care had "current" pain [1]. Another study estimated that 45–85% of elderly patients experience moderate-to-severe chronic pain [2].

Approximately 20% of older people take analgesic medications, and the majority are using these medications for greater than 6 months' duration [3]. Further, older people have the highest rate of surgical procedures and are also more likely to experience musculoskeletal pain and other chronic conditions than younger people [3]. The three most commons sites of pain in older people are the back, knee, and hip [1].

Opioids, nonsteroidal anti-inflammatory drugs (NSAIDs), acetaminophen, and adjuvant analgesic agents are reviewed.

A. J. Carinci (✉)
Division of Pain Medicine, and Pain Treatment Center, Department of Anesthesiology & Perioperative Medicine, University of Rochester Medical Center, University of Rochester School of Medicine and Dentistry, Rochester, NY, USA
e-mail: adam_carinci@urmc.rochester.edu

S. Pritzlaff
Department of Anesthesiology, Perioperative and Pain Medicine, Stanford University, Stanford, CA, USA

A. Moore
Division of Pediatric Anesthesiology, Vanderbilt University Medical Center, Nashville, TN, USA

Opioids

Overview

Opiates are derived from opium, which is harvested from the poppy *Papaver somniferum* [4]. Humans have been using this drug in various forms for thousands of years. In fact, ancient historians note that the Sumerians, inhabitants of modern-day Iraq, grew poppy plants and extracted opium from the plant's seeds at the end of the third millennium BC. Opium was termed *gil*, the word for joy, and the poppy was fittingly referred to as *hulgil*, or plant of joy [5]. Classical texts, such as Homer's *Odyssey*, also make reference to opioids as a pain-relieving substance.

Mechanism of Action/Classification

Opioid analgesics as a class can be categorized into three chemical groups: (1) synthetic phenylpiperidines (e.g., meperidine, fentanyl), (2) synthetic pseudopiperidines (e.g., methadone, propoxyphene), and (3) naturally occurring alkaloids derived directly from the poppy seed (e.g., heroin, morphine, codeine) and their semisynthetic derivatives (e.g., hydromorphone, oxycodone, oxymorphone) [6].

Opioids can also be classified as agonists, antagonists, partial agonists, and mixed agonist-antagonists. These designations are based on the particular opioid's interaction with the three main opioid receptors: mu, kappa, and delta. Opioids produce analgesia primarily through interaction with mu receptors, which are present in large quantities in the brain and spinal cord (periaqueductal gray matter and substantia gelatinosa, respectively). Activation of mu receptors also results in euphoria, respiratory depression, nausea and vomiting, and decreased gastrointestinal motility, tolerance, and dependence [4]. Activation of the kappa receptors also causes analgesia but less respiratory depression than mu receptor activation. Importantly, kappa receptor activation produces dysphoria and hallucinations rather than euphoria. Last, delta receptors produce analgesia both spinally and supraspinally [4].

Opioid receptors are coupled to G-proteins. They act both presynaptically and postsynaptically. Presynaptically, they inhibit the release of neurotransmitters, including substance P and glutamate. Postsynaptically, they can inhibit neurons by opening potassium channels that hyperpolarize the cell [4]. Opioids are complex molecules with possible action at other types of receptors including NMDA, norepinephrine, serotonin, and sodium channels. For example, some opioid medications, such as methadone, meperidine, and tramadol, have analgesic effects in part mediated by different receptors. These three drugs inhibit serotonin and norepinephrine uptake. Methadone and meperidine are antagonists of the NMDA amino acid excitatory pathway. Moreover, meperidine also blocks sodium channels and has local anesthetic properties [4].

Indications for Drug

Opioid medications are commonly used pain medicines in the elderly population on both an inpatient and outpatient basis. They have proven benefit for the treatment of acute musculoskeletal and neuropathic pain as well as cancer pain. However, studies are lacking on their efficacy for long-term treatment of chronic non-cancer pain. Randomized controlled trials have demonstrated short-term efficacy of opioids in persistent musculoskeletal pain, including osteoarthritis and low back pain, and various neuropathic pains, such as postherpetic neuralgia and diabetic peripheral neuropathy. Yet, longer-term efficacy and safety data are lacking [1].

Routes of Administration

Opioids can be administered through a variety of routes, the most common being oral, intravenous, and transdermal. There is a significant first-pass effect with the oral route (the oral to IV dose ratio is 3–1). The duration of oral opioids is prolonged by their slow absorption through the GI tract, versus intravenous administration which has faster onset and shorter duration of action. In terms of transdermal administration, the diffusion through the skin of several opioids is possible, including fentanyl and buprenorphine. Rapid titration is not possible with the transdermal route. It is particularly good for patients with stable pain and for those who cannot tolerate oral medication.

Opioids can also be administered via the rectal route (oral to rectal potency for morphine is 1:1).

Transmucosal administration is another option as well. The more lipophilic opioids are readily absorbed through buccal, nasal, or gingival mucosa. First-pass effect of the liver is avoided, and there is rapid onset of action. Buprenorphine, butorphanol, fentanyl, and sufentanil can be given via this route. While outside the scope of this chapter, opioids can also be administered IV, IM, and neuraxially.

Choice of Opioid

Choosing the proper opioid depends on a variety of patient factors, including source of the pain and whether it's acute or chronic in nature, as well as other existing comorbidities. As a start, it is important to ask patients if they have received opioids in the past and whether they have a preference. Efficacy and side effects are often patient dependent and can be idiosyncratic [4]. The best principle when prescribing opioids is to start low and titrate up (or down) in increments until optimal (maximal analgesia with acceptable side effects.) While older people tend to require lower doses than younger individuals, the effects of opioid themselves do not vary widely with age. Thus, titration of the dose based on individual response is required for people of all ages [1]. Often, pure opioid agonists are preferred over partial agonists, especially in chronic pain patients, because of their superior efficacy and easier titratability [4].

Opioids can be further subdivided into mild and strong categories. As the name implies, mild opioids (e.g., hydrocodone, oxycodone, codeine) are good for mild to moderate short-term pain. Mild opioids are often combination analgesics, containing either acetaminophen or anti-inflammatory medications. These combo products make up a significant portion of opioids prescribed by primary care physicians and pain physicians [6].

There are no primary studies relating to the use of mild opioids in older people. Some sources suggest that as an alternative, a low-dose of a more potent opioid such as morphine may be better tolerated [1]. Strong opioids include morphine, hydromorphone, and fentanyl, which are indicated when moderate-to-severe pain is no longer responsive to weak opioids.

In the treatment of prolonged pain (cancer and non-cancer), it is usually preferable to base therapy on a long-acting preparation and to use short-acting drugs from "breakthrough" pain. Long-acting opioid therapy is associated with less euphoria and dysphoria (therefore has less addictive potential) [4]. Common long-acting options include MS Contin® (morphine sulfate), OxyContin® (oxycodone), Duragesic® (fentanyl patch), and methadone. Less frequent dosing of long-acting medications is also a benefit, particularly in the elderly population who may be on a variety of other medications. A recent longitudinal study in the United States of nursing home residents found that the use of controlled-release opioids improved functional status and social engagement compared with short-acting opioids [1].

Types of Opioids

Weak Opioids

Natural opium alkaloids:

- Codeine, codeine plus acetaminophen (Tylenol #3)

  Phenanthrene derivatives

- Hydrocodone, hydrocodone plus acetaminophen (Vicodin) or aspirin (Lortab) or ibuprofen (Vicoprofen)
- Oxycodone (long-acting, OxyContin; elixir, Roxicodone), oxycodone plus acetaminophen (Percocet) or aspirin (Percodan)

  Diphenylheptane derivatives:

Propoxyphene (off market in Europe and the United States due to risk of cardiac arrhythmias)

Opioid Groups

Naturally occurring: morphine, codeine, papaverine, thebaine

Semisynthetic: heroin, dihydromorphine/morphinone, thebaine derivatives (e.g., *buprenorphine*)

Synthetic: morphinan series (e.g., *butorphanol*), *diphenylpropylamine* (e.g., *methadone*), *benzomorphan series* (e.g., *pentazocine*), *phenylpiperidine series* (e.g., *meperidine, fentanyl, remifentanil*)

Morphine

Morphine sulfate is the standard with which all other opioids are compared. It is metabolized by the liver, and 10% of the dose is excreted unchanged in the urine. The major metabolites of morphine sulfate are morphine-3-glucuronide (which is inactive) and morphine-6-glucuronide (which is more potent than morphine itself and has a longer half-life). Because these metabolites are excreted by the kidneys, patients with renal dysfunction can accumulate morphine-6-glucuronide and develop prolonged opioid effects, including respiratory depression. However, patients with liver failure tolerate morphine nearly up to the point of hepatic precoma because glucuronidation is rarely impaired [4].

Oral morphine is available in an immediate-release form and a controlled-release form.

There are no studies relating to the use of morphine specifically in older people [1]. However, it is generally observed that older people are more sensitive to the therapeutic and adverse effects of morphine. As with other opioids, dose adjustment and careful monitoring are essential when administering morphine in the older population [3].

Codeine

Codeine (a naturally occurring opium alkaloid derivative) is less potent than morphine and falls in the weak/mild opioid category. It has a similar structure to morphine, but its affinity for the mu opioid receptor is 300 times lower. It is metabolized by the liver, and its metabolites are excreted by the kidneys. Approximately 10% of codeine is demethylated to morphine by CYP2D6, giving the drug its analgesic action. Those patients with nonfunctional CYP2D6 will not be able to convert codeine to morphine, while those who have an excess of this enzyme can experience life-threatening side effects because of excessive conversion to morphine. Approximately 7–10% of Caucasians have poor CYP2D6 metabolism, whereas 1–7% have gene duplications and are classified as having ultra-rapid metabolism [7]. Some medications are CYP2D6 inhibitors, including selective serotonin reuptake inhibitors, diphenhydramine, and bupropion. Other drugs, such as rifampicin and dexamethasone, induce CYP450 isozymes and thus increase the conversion rate.

Codeine also has antitussive action which is often prescribed as a cough medication. It has decreased constipation, respiratory distress, sedation, nausea, and physical dependence compared to morphine. The number needed to treat to achieve 50% pain relief with 60 mg of codeine is 16.7, leading to its use as a combination analgesic [6].

Hydrocodone

Hydrocodone is a semisynthetic codeine derivative with analgesic and antitussive properties. It is 6–8 times more potent than codeine. It is a prodrug and undergoes CYP3A4 metabolism to noroxycodone and CYP2D6 metabolism to hydromorphone. It has a potency approximately 60% that of morphine [6]. It is commonly prescribed in combination with acetaminophen (Vicodin®). Compared with morphine, there is equivalent analgesia, respiratory depression, and physical dependency.

Hydromorphone

Hydromorphone is a semisynthetic derivative that is 5–10 times more potent than morphine. Oral dosing takes 45 min for peak effects. Unlike morphine, there is no controlled-release formulation. Hydromorphone is commonly used in both cancer and non-cancer pain, although it has not been specifically studied in older people [1]. It is considered to be safer than morphine for use in patients with renal dysfunction.

Oxycodone

Oxycodone is a semisynthetic opioid agonist. It's a thebaine derivative with a similar profile and 1.5 times the potency of morphine. It has an established role in the treatment of acute pain.

Ten percent of oxycodone is metabolized to oxymorphone, which has up to five times the affinity for the mu receptor compared with morphine. The most abundant metabolite of oxycodone is noroxycodone, which has weak affinity for mu receptors. Oxycodone may also have analgesic activity at the kappa receptor, which explains why it is useful in patients not responsive to morphine [6].

Oxycodone is available in many formulations including controlled (OxyContin®)- and immediate-release tablets as well as elixir. It is also available in parenteral, rectal, and intranasal forms. It is commonly prescribed as part of a combination analgesic with acetaminophen, nonsteroidal anti-inflammatory drugs, and aspirin. Oxycodone is a useful substitute for morphine in the elderly who are sensitive to morphine-6-glucuronide and morphine-induced sedation and mental status change (MGH Pain, p. 121). Compared with morphine, it has slightly more potent analgesia and incidence of side effects [6].

Recent studies have investigated the safety and efficacy of longer-term oxycodone use in the treatment of chronic nociceptive and neuropathic pain. While these studies have included older people (over 65 years), knowledge of the specific efficacy and tolerability of oxycodone in the elderly is limited. The pharmacokinetics of oxycodone in younger people suggests that it is a suitable opioid for use in the elderly, particularly because of its relatively short half-life and predictable dose-response curve [3].

In hospitalized elderly patients, oxycodone is a suitable choice of opioid because of its relatively fewer pharmacological issues such as dose adjustment with decreased renal function and few drug-drug interactions [3]. A study showed the elimination half-life of oxycodone in patients with renal impairment was prolonged by 1 h [2]. It is important to note that, in older patients, oral oxycodone is associated with significantly more constipation than transdermal fentanyl [1].

Meperidine

Meperidine is metabolized to normeperidine, which has a half-life of 15–20 h and is eliminated by both the kidney and the liver. It can accumulate in people with renal or hepatic function. Normeperidine is toxic, and large doses can cause tremors, muscle twitches, dilated pupils, hyperactive reflexes, and convulsions. Meperidine should not be combined with MAOs. It has vagolytic activities and is the only opioid that may produce tachycardia, so additional caution should be exercised. Besides acting on opioid receptors, meperidine also has weak local anesthetic activities. In addition to serving as an analgesic, meperidine is also effective for the treatment of postoperative shivering.

Meperidine is often avoided, especially for long-term use, because of the possibility of normeperidine toxicity and because the drug has euphoric side effects and high abuse potential. Meperidine is not included in pain management guidelines.

Levorphanol

Levorphanol (levo-3-hydroxy-N-methylmorphinan) is a morpinium drug that is pharmacologically similar to morphine. It was originally synthesized as a pharmacological alternative to morphine more than 40 years ago.

Levorphanol produces analgesia via its interactions with mu, delta, and kappa opioid receptors. Levorphanol is also an N-methyl-D-aspartate (NMDA) receptor antagonist, and it may inhibit the uptake of norepinephrine and serotonin [8]. Levorphanol undergoes glucuronidation in the liver, and the glucuronidated products are excreted in the kidney. Levorphanol can be given orally, intravenously, and subcutaneously. It is 4–8 times as potent as morphine and has a longer half-life. Of note, it is associated with less nausea and vomiting than morphine.

Methadone

Methadone was developed in Germany in 1937 and was later introduced into the United States in 1947 by Eli Lilly and Company. It is the only opioid with prolonged activity not achieved by controlled-release formulation. In addition to its mu and delta opioid receptor agonist effect, it is an NMDA inhibitor and also an inhibitor of serotonin and norepinephrine reuptake. It is a good option for patients with refractory difficult-to-control chronic pain and is also used for detoxification or maintenance treatment of opioid addicts.

Methadone has biphasic elimination. The analgesic action equates to the alpha elimination phase, which typically lasts 6–8 h, and a long beta elimination phase that ranges from 30 to 60 h, which corresponds with its ability to prevent withdrawals and cravings. Thus, sedation and respiratory depression can outlast the analgesic action. This biphasic pattern helps to explain why methadone is needed every 4–8 h for analgesia but only once a day for opioid maintenance therapy. The oral to parenteral dose ratio is 2:1.

There is high variability in steady-state plasma levels in different individuals. It undergoes N-demethylation by the liver cytochrome P-450 enzymes (this activity can vary widely in different individuals). Multiple drug interactions can occur, especially with antivirals and antibiotics. In patients taking methadone, QTc interval must be monitored for signs of prolongation. Rapid titration of methadone is not advisable, so this drug should be reserved for patients with stable chronic pain [4].

Fentanyl

Fentanyl is a potent and highly lipophilic semisynthetic opioid agonist (phenylpiperidine compound) that rapidly penetrates the blood-brain barrier, resulting in prompt onset of analgesia. It is 50–80 times as potent as morphine and can be used as an analgesic or anesthetic. Fentanyl undergoes extensive oxidative metabolism to norfentanyl, an inactive metabolite, which is subsequently excreted by the kidneys. Its metabolism is mediated by CYP3A4.

Due to high first-pass effect, fentanyl is unsuitable for oral administration. It can be given via the parenteral, transdermal, and buccal routes. It is most commonly given as a transdermal patch for the treatment of chronic pain. After initial application of the patch, a depot of fentanyl forms in the cutaneous layers of the skin, with subsequent absorption into the circulation (maximum blood levels may take 12 h to be reached, after which analgesia persists for up to 72 h). The transdermal route bypasses the liver resulting in fairly constant blood levels, resulting in a convenient and comfortable system [4]. A meta-analysis comparing transdermal fentanyl and slow-release oral morphine found that fentanyl produced a significantly greater reduction in "right now" pain ratings than morphine in patients with chronic non-cancer pain. This reduction was less apparent in subgroup analyses in patients over 60 years and in patients with low BMIs [3].

Because rapid titration is not possible, transdermal fentanyl should not be used in patients who are opioid naïve due to the risk of excessive pharmacological effects and toxicity. It is not recommended for use in acute settings due to the delayed onset of action and risk of respiratory depression. The transdermal route offers a number of advantages in the treatment of chronic pain. Steady drug concentrations can be achieved in a noninvasive manner, and the challenges of oral administration, such as low oral bioavailability, swallowing difficulties, nausea, and vomiting, can be avoided [3]. It is also preferred in the elderly population for reasons of compliance and convenience, as the patch only needs to be changed every 48–72 h [2]. Another benefit is that transdermal fentanyl may be associated with less constipation than oral oxycodone in older people [1].

Despite the stable pharmacokinetic profile of transdermal fentanyl, a high degree of inter-patient variability in concentration-time profiles has been reported [3]. For example, drug permeation through the skin is influenced by many factors such as application site, skin temperature, sweat gland function, and skin integrity. However, the rate-limiting membrane in the fentanyl patch helps to minimize the impact of these factors [3]. Fentanyl may exhibit a larger volume of distribution and longer half-life in older people, given the changes in body composition that accompany aging. For example, age-related decreases in liver blood flow would be expected to result in lower hepatic clearance [3].

Buprenorphine

Buprenorphine is a highly lipophilic, semisynthetic opioid with partial activity at the mu receptor and very little activity at the kappa and delta receptor. It has high affinity but low intrinsic activity at the mu receptor, which results in a pharmacologic ceiling effect. Given this, it is sometimes chosen because of its low potential for abuse and respiratory depression. It has been increasingly used in the treatment of chronic pain in the elderly due to the availability of a transdermal delivery system that provides sustained analgesia over an extended period. However, there is limited data for its use in older people. Buprenorphine is also used as maintenance therapy in patients being treated for opioid dependence. Suboxone® (four parts buprenorphine, one part naloxone) is a combination drug used for office-based treatment of opioid dependence/addiction. The naloxone is added as a deterrent for injecting this medication intravenously.

One potential problem for patients on buprenorphine is how to address the treatment of "breakthrough" pain with immediate-release opioid agonists, which may theoretically be antagonized by buprenorphine, thus limiting its effectiveness. However, a number of studies have demonstrated that the administration of morphine and other opioids for the management of breakthrough pain is both safe and effective for patients on transdermal buprenorphine [3]. Several studies have shown that the partial agonism of buprenorphine gives a ceiling effect for respiratory depression, but no clinically relevant analgesic ceiling [2]. However, in a study by Griessinger et al. comprising 13,179 patients, 49.6% of subjects required concomitant analgesics during buprenorphine treatment [2].

An uncontrolled, observational study with 93 elderly patients concluded that transdermal buprenorphine was effective and safe in the treatment of elderly patients with nonmalignant pain. They also noted that transdermal buprenorphine did not influence cognitive and behavioral functions in elderly patients [2]. Transdermal buprenorphine patches only need to be changed every 7 days, thus reducing administration time and allowing for ease of use, a benefit for the elderly population.

While buprenorphine is metabolized in part by CYP3A4, inhibitors or inducers of this enzyme are not expected to cause significant alteration of buprenorphine metabolism or effects. Moreover, age does not have a significant effect on buprenorphine pharmacokinetics after transdermal administration [3]. Several studies have shown that buprenorphine is not altered in elderly patients with renal impairment [2].

Tramadol

Tramadol is a synthetic centrally acting analgesic with a unique mode of action. It has weak opioid activity at the mu, delta, and kappa receptors, with a 20-fold preference for the mu receptor. In addition, it has norepinephrine and serotonin reuptake inhibition. It is indicated for mild-to-moderate pain but can also be used to treat severe pain (in combination with other analgesics). It has a lower potential for addiction and respiratory depression compared to other opioids, making it a popular choice [1]. Its affinity for the mu opioid receptor is approximately 10 times weaker than codeine and 6000 times weaker than morphine [6]. It is available in an immediate-release and controlled-release form. It has been available in Germany since 1977 but was only released in the United States in 1995.

Tramadol is metabolized by the liver CYP enzyme system and is excreted by the kidneys (90%) and feces (10%). Biotransformation in the liver creates 23 metabolites (M1 is the primary metabolite). Individuals with a mutation in the CYP2D6 isoenzyme may cause inadequate analgesia in poor metabolizers [6].

There are no primary studies relating to the use of tramadol in older people. A prospective, age-controlled study suggests older people require 20% less tramadol than younger adults, although the pharmacokinetics remains unaffected by age [1]. Tramadol may reduce the seizure threshold and is contraindicated in patients with a history of seizures and should be used with caution in patients taking other serotonergic drugs. Adjustments are required in patients with hepatic and renal failure. Compared with morphine and other traditional opioids, tramadol has a more favorable side effect profile, although up to 16.8% of patients taking tramadol for chronic pain may experience side effects [6].

Tapentadol

Tapentadol has a dual mechanism of action as an opioid agonist and noradrenaline reuptake inhibitor. It was recently approved in the United States (2008) for the treatment of moderate-to-severe chronic pain. Because of a lack of empiric knowledge, the use of tapentadol is not recommended in frail elderly persons.

Age-Specific Considerations

Respiratory depression is the most feared of the opioid side effects. This can lead to hypoxia, apnea, and even death. However, this is much more likely to occur when opioids are used for the treatment of acute rather than chronic pain or in opioid-naïve patients. The opioid titration principle is particularly important for avoiding this side effect [4].

Nausea, vomiting, and constipation are the most frequently reported adverse side effects. Nausea and vomiting occur mainly at the beginning of the treatment with opioids and can be avoided by slow titration to the effective dose and antiemetics if necessary. When opioid-induced nausea does occur, it can be treated by reducing the opioid dose, trialing another opioid, or giving an antiemetic [4].

Constipation is one of most common side effects of both acute and chronic opioid use. Prophylactic stimulant laxative therapy is recommended in nearly all patients using chronic opioids.

Central side effects of opioids include drowsiness and dizziness. Sedation is a common adverse side effect but mainly occurs in the beginning of treatment. This may be associated with an increased incidence of falls and fractures in the elderly population. Opioids can also produce peripheral vasodilation, which may lead to orthostatic hypotension. This is important in older individuals because of the increased risk of falls. Mental confusion and hallucinations occur frequently in the elderly, especially those who are opioid naïve [1]. In patients taking stable doses of opioids, cognitive function is relatively unaffected, but it may be impaired for up to a week after a dose increase [1].

Common side effects, such as sedation, nausea, and vomiting, are often worse around opioid initiation or dose escalation and may resolve after 2 or 3 days. However, constipation does not readily improve and should be managed with prophylactic laxative therapy unless medically contraindicated [1]. To help manage adverse effects during opioid therapy, opioid rotation can be used to address the problem of tolerance, achieve increased analgesic response, and minimize side effects [2].

Age is an important predictor of opioid-related harm. Patients over 60 years of age have a two- to eightfold increased risk of respiratory depression and falls and fractures [3].

Dosing Considerations

Renal and Hepatic Disease
For patients with hepatic and renal disease, concerns arise over decreased metabolism and elimination. The metabolites of opioids are mainly excreted by the kidneys. Active metabolites of morphine and codeine, especially morphine-6-glucuronide, may accumulate in patients with renal dysfunction. Meperidine administration can lead to the accumulation of normeperidine, causing CNS excitation with tremors or seizures.

In terms of liver function, methadone administration with drugs that inhibit CYP 3A4 enzymes may result in increased plasma concentrations of methadone. Conversely, inducers of CYP 3A4 or CYP2D6 enzymes may result in withdrawal symptoms. Fentanyl and buprenorphine are metabolized by CYP3A4 into inactive metabolites. Morphine, hydromorphone, and oxymorphone are not metabolized by CYP but are metabolized UGT enzymes. Opioid analgesics, like any medication, may be metabolized by the CYP drug-metabolizing enzyme system 2D6. Genetic polymorphism of CYP2D6 may lead to variability in enzyme breakdown and clinical effectiveness of the medication. Deficiency of CYP2D6 may be seen in whites (7%) and those of Asian descent (1%) [6].

Respiratory Disease
For patients with respiratory disease (e.g., emphysema, kyphoscoliosis, extreme obesity), opioids should be prescribed with caution. Opioids that release histamine, such as morphine, may precipitate bronchospasm, especially in asthmatics. Moreover, suppression of cough reflex may be dangerous in patients with copious sections (e.g., pneumonia, bronchiectasis, post-thoracotomy) [4]. Opioids should not be administered for those with acute respiratory depression and severe COPD.

Drug Interactions.
The elderly are at risk for drug interactions. For example, interactions between opioids and antiretroviral agents may change plasma concentrations of methadone, buprenorphine, morphine, and fentanyl. Avoid concurrent use of alcohol and opioids.

Summary Points

Opioids are among the most effective analgesic options available, which is logical considering natural analgesic states are mediated by endogenous opioids and that opioid medications produce pain relief by binding to these natural receptors. Opioids have demonstrated efficacy in acute and cancer pain, but data on chronic pain are lacking. Elderly patients with moderate-to-severe pain may be good candidates for opioid therapy, particularly if they are experiencing functional impairment or reduced quality of life. Patients with stable chronic pain should be managed with transdermal or controlled-release oral formulations, as opposed to immediate-release options. Opioids must be titrated carefully on a patient by patient basis as there is a wide degree of variability. Moreover, physicians must monitor for side effects and should also prescribe prophylactic therapy (e.g., laxatives and anti-nausea medications). Opioid rotation can also be considered for patients requiring escalating doses of a particular opioid medication [1].

Van Ojik et al. conducted a literature search on opioid use in the elderly. They concluded that no differentiation can be made between the appropriateness of buprenorphine, fentanyl, hydromorphone, morphine, and oxycodone for use in elderly patients. Methadone has strong negative considerations in the treatment of chronic pain in the frail elderly. Methadone has high drug-drug interaction potential and is associated with prolongation of the QT interval and a potential risk of accumulation due to a long elimination half-life. It is also difficult to titrate because of its large inter-individual variability in pharmacokinetics.

A discussion of opioid use for pain management is not complete without mentioning the opioid crisis. A decision to use opioids to treat chronic pain includes an evaluation for addiction and misuse of opioids. See Chapter "Assessing and Managing Addiction Risk in Older Adults with Pain" for a discussion of addiction and misuse in the elderly.

Nonsteroidal Anti-inflammatory Drugs

Overview

Nonsteroidal anti-inflammatory drugs (NSAIDs) are a chemically diverse group of medications that have analgesic, antipyretic, and anti-inflammatory properties. They are among the most commonly prescribed drugs in the world, particularly among the aging population. Perhaps the best known NSAID is acetylsalicylic acid (ASA), better known as aspirin. Derived from salicylic acid, a compound originally isolated from the bark of the willow plant, aspirin has continued to have a presence worldwide since Bayer Pharmaceuticals started manufacturing it over 100 years ago. Aspirin set the stage for the subsequent discovery of other chemically diverse drugs with a similar action. John Robert Vane, an English pharmacologist, was the principle investigator who elucidated the mechanism of action of NSAIDs, receiving the Nobel Prize for this work in 1982. Despite the ubiquitous use of these medications in the outpatient and acute care settings, healthcare providers must be aware of the limitations and dangers of NSAIDS in their aging patients.

Mechanism of Action

NSAIDS are inhibitors of cyclooxygenase (COX), the enzyme that catalyzes the formation of prostaglandins (PG) and thromboxane from arachidonic acid. Arachidonic acid is a polyunsaturated fatty acid that forms the basis for all tissues in mammals. When tissue injury occurs, arachidonic acid is released, and an inflammatory cascade ensues. Its 20-carbon structure forms the template for all eicosanoids, the main signaling molecules involved with inflammation. Eicosanoids include PGs, thromboxanes, hydroxy acids, and leukotrienes.

COX consists of two isoenzymes, cyclooxygenase-1 (COX-1) and cyclooxygenase-2 (COX-2). NSAIDs competitively inhibit COX nonselectively, whereas aspirin is an irreversible inhibitor of the enzyme. COX-1 is a constitutively expressed enzyme and plays a role in regulating many normal physiologic processes in the body. Perhaps one of its most important roles and of significant importance with elderly populations is maintenance of the gastric lining in the stomach. Prostaglandins play a vital role in protecting and maintaining the integrity of the gastric mucosa from damage from the acidic environment. When nonselective COX-1/COX-2 inhibitors (commonly ibuprofen and aspirin) are used regularly, ulcers of the stomach or duodenum can develop. COX-2 is facultatively expressed, mediating inflammation, fever, and pain. Inhibition of this enzyme produces desirable effects of NSAIDs.

Despite good efficacy, NSAIDs must be used with caution in older people because of a high risk of potentially serious and life-threatening side effects, as prostaglandins have a pivotal role in the normal human physiological functions of the GI tract and renal and cardiovascular systems, among others. NSAIDs have been implicated in up to a quarter of hospital admissions due to adverse drug reactions in older people [9].

Pharmacokinetics

NSAIDs are weak acids with pKa values typically lower than 5. Under normal physiologic conditions, these anti-inflammatory agents will be present in the body mostly in the ionized form. The majority of NSAID preparations are oral formulations, and the peak plasma concentrations are typically reached after 2–4 h. All NSAIDs are lipid-soluble, highly bound to plasma proteins (>99%), mainly albumin. Aspirin binds to plasma proteins to a lesser degree, typically in the 75–90% range depending on the dose. There is no conclusive evidence that sodium bicarbonate given with aspirin (buffered aspirin) results in a faster onset of action, greater peak intensity, or longer analgesic effect. Aspirin available in buffered effervescent preparations, however, undergoes a more rapid systemic absorption and achieves higher plasma concentrations than the corresponding tablet formulations. These effervescent preparations also cause less gastrointestinal irritation. The implications of protein binding are significant since hypoalbuminemia, a condition with increased prevalence in the elderly, can increase the free plasma concentration of NSAIDs. Elimination occurs primarily by hepatic biotransformation, although renal excretion also plays a minor role as well. Table 1 outlines commonly prescribed NSAIDs.

Table 1 Nonsteroidal anti-inflammatory drugs[a]

Name	Class	Dosing	Considerations
Aspirin	Nonselective COX enzyme inhibitor	Max. dose, 4000 mg/d in divided doses	Salicylate levels can be monitored
Celecoxib (Celebrex®)	COX 2 enzyme inhibitor selective	Max. dose: 200 mg bid	Less platelet inhibition and gastric toxicity
Diclofenac	COX inhibition	Max dose 150 mg/d	Metabolized through the liver primarily CYP2C9; available in gel form
Diflunisal	COX inhibition	Max dose 1000 mg/day in divided doses	Dose may need to be decreased in small patients and frail patients
Etodolac	COX inhibition	Max dose 1000 mg/d in divided doses	Use with caution in people with renal disease
Ibuprofen (Motrin®)	Nonselective COX enzyme inhibitor	Max dose 2400 mg/d in divided doses	Available over the counter; be sure to ask about over-the-counter pain medications; can cause confusion in the elderly
Indomethacin (Indocin®)	COX inhibition	Max dose 150 mg/d in divided doses	Dose may need to be decreased in small patients and frail patients
Ketoprofen	COX inhibition	Max dose 225 mg/d in divided doses	Available in cream preparation
Ketorolac (Toradol®)	COX inhibition	Max dose 60 mg/d in divided doses	Available in intravenous and intramuscular preparations; DO NOT use more than 5 days secondary to toxicity
Nabumetone (Relafen®)	Partial COX 2 selective	Max dose 200 mg/day	Avoid max dose for prolonged periods
Naproxen (Aleve®, Naprosyn®)	COX inhibition	Max dose 1000 mg/day in divided doses	Available over the counter; be sure to ask about over-the-counter pain medications; can cause confusion in the elderly
Oxaprozin (Daypro®)	COX inhibition	Max dose 1200 mg/d in divided doses	Same side effect profile as all NSAIDs
Piroxicam (Feldene®)	COX inhibition	Max dose 20 mg/d	Can use in single daily dose
Salsalate	COX inhibition	Max dose 3000 md/d in divided doses	Hydrolyzed to aspirin in small intestine
Sulindac (Clinoril®)	COX inhibition	Max dose 400 mg/d in divided doses	Same side effect profile as all NSAID

[a]All NSAIDs carrying a black box warning except aspirin; these medications if used should be at the lowest effective dose and for the shortest duration secondary to the side effects of the medications

Indications for Use

NSAIDs are among the most common medications for the treatment of a variety of pain complaints in the elderly including musculoskeletal and inflammatory pain conditions. Osteoarthritis, lower back pain, and muscle strain have a high prevalence in this population. In general, over-the-counter agents have a good safety profile if prescribed appropriately. With that said, particular caution must be exercised when considering NSAID therapy for individuals with low creatinine clearance, gastropathy, cardiovascular disease, or intravascularly depleted states such as congestive heart failure [10].

Routes of Administration

NSAIDs are available for oral administration. Ketorolac is available for intravenous administration. Several NSAIDs are available in a gel or cream.

Considerations for Older Adults

When considering NSAIDs as part of a treatment regimen, providers must weigh the potential risks of these medications based on a patient's clinical condition. All commonly used NSAIDs are on Beers list of inappropriate medications for older adults. Compiled by the American Geriatrics Society, the Beers Criteria are intended for use in all ambulatory and institutional settings of care for populations aged 65 and older in the United States. The intentions of the criteria include improving the selection of prescription drugs by clinicians and patients, evaluating patterns of drug use within populations, and educating clinicians and patients on proper drug usage [10].

COX-2 inhibitors like celecoxib are of particular interest to many patients, as they were initially touted at the NSAIDs with a minimal side effect profile given their selectivity. Although the incidence of gastrointestinal complications is decreased with these drugs, they appear to increase the risk of cardiovascular side effects, including an increased risk of myocardial infarction.

Even short-term use of NSAIDS has been considered unacceptable in older adults with diabetes, impaired kidney function, or taking medications that may impair kidney function (diuretics, angiotensin-converting enzyme inhibitors) or metformin. The patient's risk factors for toxicities and adverse drug reactions (including renal insufficiency, congestive heart failure, hypertension, or concomitant medications such as warfarin use) and recent history of NSAID exposure should be reviewed before administering or prescribing NSAIDs [11]. NSAIDs have been implicated in up to a quarter (23.5%) of hospital admissions due to adverse drug reactions in older people [9].

Perhaps the greatest risk to older adults taking NSAIDs is the high incidence of drug-drug interactions. The average adult over the age of 65 takes multiple medications for conditions such as hypertension and diabetes. It is critical that primary care providers frequently update and reconcile a patient's medication profile. For example, indomethacin is known to interfere with the action of many antihypertensives including atenolol, propranolol, prazosin, captopril, and thiazide diuretics. It also blunts the diuretic response of furosemide, triamterene, and

Table 2 Common side effects of NSAIDs in older adults

Gastrointestinal effects	GI toxicity: bleeding and ulceration Increased likelihood of adverse GI effects when an NSAID is co-administered with low-dose aspirin or warfarin
Central nervous effects	Tinnitus or deafness can occur if toxic levels are achieved. Toxic manifestations are directly related to free drug levels, which vary inversely with albumin levels. The most frequently implicated class of drugs in hypersensitivity-induced aseptic meningitis
Renal effects	Renal vasoconstriction and increased tubular sodium reabsorption can lead to fluid retention and possible exacerbation of congestive cardiac failure Can contribute to worsening of chronic renal failure, particularly in patients taking diuretics or angiotensin-converting enzyme inhibitors
Cardiovascular effects	Reported modest increases in blood pressure. Older adults taking antihypertensive agents at greatest risk for complications All NSAIDs, including COX-2 inhibitors, may increase the risk of cardiovascular thrombotic events, myocardial infarction, and stroke

spironolactone. Salicylates in therapeutic doses have been shown to enhance the effects of oral hypoglycemic agents, especially chlorpropamide. Table 2 outlines the risks of NSAIDs.

Acetaminophen

Overview

Acetaminophen, chemically named N-acetyl-p-aminophenol, is a common analgesic and antipyretic similar to those of aspirin. It is commonly known elsewhere in the world by its international nonproprietary name, paracetamol. Unlike NSAIDs, acetaminophen possesses very weak anti-inflammatory properties. Acetaminophen is part of the class of drugs known as "aniline analgesics," the only drug still manufactured in this class. Acetaminophen, or paracetamol, is the active metabolite of phenacetin, a previously sold and highly popular analgesic and antipyretic. Phenacetin was discontinued in the United States in 1983 due to concerns of carcinogenic and renal toxic properties. Contrary to its precursor, paracetamol is not considered carcinogenic at therapeutic doses. Acetaminophen remains a popular choice for pain control in the aging population because of its more favorable side effect profile as compared to NSAIDs, namely, its lack of GI side effects.

Mechanism of Action

Acetaminophen has analgesic and antipyretic properties similar to those of aspirin. Its mechanism of action remains a point of debate and is still a focus of research. The antipyretic effect probably occurs because of direct action on the hypothalamic heat-regulating centers via the inhibiting action of endogenouspyrogen. Its analgesic properties are less clear, although recent data suggests that it acts on serotonergic pathways. Other proposed mechanisms include the inhibition of cyclooxygenase

(COX), specifically COX-2. Although equipotent to aspirin in inhibiting central prostaglandin synthesis, acetaminophen has no significant peripheral prostaglandin synthetase inhibition. Doses of 650 mg have been shown to be more effective than doses of 300 mg, but little additional benefit is seen at doses above 1000 mg, indicating a possible ceiling effect [4]. It is this lack of peripheral activity is the reason why acetaminophen is not a great choice for inflammatory conditions.

Acetaminophen is completely and rapidly absorbed when given orally. Peak serum concentrations are typically achieved within 2 h in most individuals. About 90% of acetaminophen is hepatically metabolized to sulfate and glucuronide conjugates for renal excretion, with a small amount secreted unchanged in the urine. Rectal administration of the drug results in significant bioavailability of the drug. In general, rectal dosing is 80% of the oral dose, and the rate of absorption is slower, with maximum plasma concentration achieved about 2–3 h after administration.

Intravenous acetaminophen has recently been available in the United States since its approval by the Food and Drug Administration in 2010. The main advantage of the IV form is its rapid onset of action, approximately 15–30 min after administration. The peak analgesic effect is reached at approximately 1 h. The maximum blood concentration (Cmax) is higher than with oral or rectal administration; however, it is important to note that the Cmax with IV acetaminophen (29 mcg/mL) remains far below the 150 mcg/ mL concentration considered potentially hepatotoxic. Unlike oral or rectal preparations, there is no first-pass metabolism of this IV form. Thus, the liver exposure is minimized, likely making this a better choice for older patients with chronic liver disease.

Indications for Use
Acetaminophen is a good choice for lower back pain, osteoarthritis, and generalized musculoskeletal pain. It is recommended by the American Geriatrics Society as a first-line agent for mild ongoing and persistent pain, with increased dosing if pain relief is not satisfactory (up to 4 mg/24 h) before moving onto a stronger alternative [12].

Route of Administration
Acetaminophen is available for oral and intravenous administration.

Considerations for Older Adults
Adverse effects are rare, and acetaminophen use is not associated with significant GI side effects, adverse effects on the renal and central nervous systems, or cardiovascular toxicity. There is increasing concern regarding the hepatic effects of prolonged use of the maximum recommended doses of acetaminophen [1]. Chronic acetaminophen use and the potential dangers of hepatic toxicity are well known by physicians and healthcare providers. It is critical that patients and their home caregivers are educated about the maximum daily dose of acetaminophen, typically 4 grams/24 h. Many patients may take more than the recommended dose because they are unaware of the potential risks of what they perceive as a "safe" drug. They may also be unaware that acetaminophen is found as an ingredient in numerous

over-the-counter agents, including cold remedies, which may lead them to exceed the recommended maximum dose unintentionally [13]. Transient elevations of alanine aminotransferase have been observed in patients taking acetaminophen chronically, although these elevations do not translate into liver failure or hepatic dysfunction when maximum recommended doses are avoided [14]. In general, it is recommended that the maximum dose of acetaminophen is reduced 50–75% in patients with hepatic insufficiency or history of alcohol abuse [12].

Adjuvant Analgesic Agents: Tricyclic Antidepressants and Serotonin-Norepinephrine Reuptake Inhibitors

Overview

Adjuvant analgesic agents are a category of medications that are effective as sole agents or in combination to treat painful syndromes primarily neuropathic agents. This category was originally used in the cancer pain literature, although the term is now used regardless of pain etiology, and describes drugs that were developed for other indications and then found to have analgesic effects [1]. Adjuvant drugs include antidepressants, antiepileptics, and corticosteroids.

Mechanism of Action

Antidepressants Tricyclic antidepressants (TCA), serotonin-norepinephrine reuptake inhibitors (SNRI), noradrenergic and specific serotonergic antidepressants (NSSAs), and selective serotonin reuptake inhibitors have been studied. These agents work through multiple pathways in the central nervous system. Their main mechanism of action involves reinforcement of the descending inhibitory pathways by increasing the amount of norepinephrine and serotonin in the synaptic cleft at both supraspinal and spinal levels. TCAs are the prototypical antidepressant compounds for the treatment of pain and are by far the most studied.

TCAs inhibit presynaptic reuptake of serotonin and norepinephrine and block cholinergic, adrenergic, histaminergic, and sodium channels. Voltage-gated sodium channels have been implicated in many types of chronic pain syndromes because these channels play a fundamental role in the excitability of neurons in the central and peripheral nervous systems. By blocking sodium channels, TCAs have been shown to be effective in the suppression of persistent pain signal [16]. SNRIs and NSSAs work in a similar fashion to tricyclics, increasing levels of both serotonin and norepinephrine, but lack many of the adverse side effects associated with TCAs. Most SNRIs including venlafaxine and duloxetine are several folds more selective for serotonin over norepinephrine. SSRIs only affect serotonin. Drugs that affect both systems have greater analgesic effect.

TCAs are well absorbed orally and are bound to serum proteins. This class of drugs undergoes rapid first-pass hepatic metabolism, but they have relatively long elimination half-lives of 1–4 days due to their lipophilic nature. Diseases that affect serum proteins or decrease liver function can alter the serum levels of these drugs.

These drugs are excreted in the urine and feces. SNRIs are highly variable in the time to peak plasma concentration and elimination half-lives. For both venlafaxine and duloxetine, elimination is both renal and hepatic; thus, dose adjustment is needed in the setting of renal or hepatic insufficiency.

Indications for Use
TCAs have good evidence showing positive results in the treatment of painful diabetic neuropathy, postherpetic neuralgia (PHN), painful polyneuropathy, and postmastectomy pain. It is important to note that these medications have not shown significant benefit in phantom limb pain, neuropathic cancer pain, chronic lumbar root pain, chemotherapy-induced neuropathy, and human immunodeficiency virus (HIV) neuropathy [15].

SNRIs have similar indications for the treatment of chronic pain as compared to TCAs but, overall, tend to have a better side effect profile in older adults. The SNRIs (duloxetine, venlafaxine) are particularly effective in the treatment of various neuropathic pain conditions and fibromyalgia, with a better side effect profile than the tricyclic antidepressants [12].

Routes of Administration
TCAs and SNRIs are available for oral administration.

Considerations for Older Adults
The biggest considerations for the use of TCAs and SNRIs in older adults are side effects. Table 2 outlines the side effects of the common medications used. TCAs are on the Beers list secondary to the anticholinergic effects of these medications (Table 3).

Antiepileptics

Overview
As a group, antiepileptic drugs inhibit ectopic neuronal signal generation and propagation from an epileptogenic focus by inhibiting various ion channels (most commonly sodium and calcium channels). Abnormal signal generation and propagation seen in the central nervous system during epileptic episodes are similar to what's observed in chronic pain states – especially chronic neuropathic pain where we see pathological signal generation from injured nerves against relatively benign stimuli or no stimuli at all. These heightened neuronal activities underlie clinical presentation of epilepsy, hyperalgesia, and allodynia. Therefore, the use of antiepileptic agents in chronic pain management was proposed.

Sodium channel blocker medications include phenytoin (Dilantin®), carbamazepine (Tegretol®), oxcarbazepine (Trileptal®), lamotrigine (Lamictal®), valproic acid (Depakote®), topiramate (Topamax®), and levetiracetam (Keppra®). Carbamazepine, oxcarbazepine, and topiramate are the three most commonly used sodium channel-blocking antiepileptic agents in chronic pain.

Table 3 Overview of common TCAs and SNRIs: dosing and side effects

Medication	Class	Dosing	Considerations and side effects
Amitriptyline	TCA, tertiary amine	25–150 mg qhs	Significant risk of adverse effects in older patients. Anticholinergic effects (visual, urinary, gastrointestinal); cardiovascular effects (orthostasis, atrioventricular blockade) Older persons rarely tolerate doses greater than 75 to 100 mg per day
Nortriptyline/ desipramine	TCA, secondary amine	10–25 mg qd (max 150 mg)	Less sedation and orthostasis compared with amitriptyline Should be used cautiously in older patients with cardiac arrhythmia and those prone to psychic activation or agitation
Trazodone	TCA	75–300 mg qhs	Potential priapism; counsel male patients Sedating effects similar to amitriptyline but minimal cardiac, anticholinergic, and orthostatic side effects
Venlafaxine	SNRI	37.5–225 mg qd	Dose-related increases in blood pressure and heart rate GI side effects, increased HR and BP, ECG abnormalities (rare)
Duloxetine	SNRI	30–120 mg qd	Monitor blood pressure, as increases in BP are possible CNS disturbances: dizziness, cognitive effects, and memory Rare nausea and hepatoxicity

Calcium channel blocker medications include gabapentin (Neurontin®), pregabalin (Lyrica®), zonisamide (Zonegran®), and ziconotide (Prialt®). Gabapentin and pregabalin are the two most commonly used calcium channel-blocking antiepileptic agents in chronic pain.

Mechanisms of Action
As mentioned above, the development of chronic pain state from a tissue injury involves heightened neuronal activation. This occurs via complex genetic-level modification resulting in increased ion channel placement (including both sodium and calcium channels) leading to neuronal membrane hyper-excitation and ectopy generation. Both sodium and calcium channel blockers inhibit ectopy generation and its signal propagation.

Indications for Drug
Antiepileptic drugs have been used for neuropathic pain for decades. The older medications have been used off label, and the newer medications have Food and Drug Administration (FDA)-approved uses in neuropathic pain. Most of the medications have one FDA approval but are used in other neuropathic conditions.

Routes of Administration
All antiepileptic drugs used in chronic pain management are administered orally. Medications like phenytoin and carbamazepine can be given IV route. Ziconotide is given intrathecally.

Age-Specific Considerations

All antiepileptics can cause sedation and somnolence in the elderly. See Table 4 for details about the use of each medication, FDA-approved uses, side effects, and age-specific considerations.

Table 4 Antiepileptic medications used to treat pain

Medication	Indication/use	FDA	Dosing	Considerations/side effects
Carbamazepine (Tegretol®)	Trigeminal or glossopharyngeal neuralgia	Yes	100 mg tid; max. dose 1200 mg/day; follow drug levels	Hyponatremia, pancytopenia (need periodic blood test), sedation, somnolence; if renal or hepatic impairment does not give loading dose to start medication
	Diabetic neuropathy, postherpetic neuropathy, poststroke pain syndrome	No		
Gabapentin (Neurontin®)	Post-herpetic neuralgia	Yes	100–300 mg. qHS; daily max. 3600 mg	Fatigue; gradually increasing dose can minimize fatigue
	Diabetic neuropathy, fibromyalgia, neuropathic pain, postoperative adjunct, restless leg syndrome	No		
Lamotrigine (Lamictal®)	Second-line agent for trigeminal neuralgia especially for those carbamazepine and/or oxcarbazepine is not effective	No	25–50 mg qHS to start; max. dose 500 mg	Rash can develop if used with lamotrigine; Stevens-Johnson syndrome
Oxcarbazepine (Trileptal®)	Trigeminal or glossopharyngeal neuralgia	Yes	600 mg. bid to start; daily max. dose 1800 mg	Hyponatremia; does not cause pancytopenia
	Diabetic neuropathy, postherpetic neuropathy, poststroke pain syndrome	No		
Pregabalin (Lyrica®)	Fibromyalgia, diabetic neuropathy, spinal cord injury neuropathy, postherpetic neuralgia	Yes	50 mg. tid or 75 mg. bid; daily max. dose 600 mg	Somnolence, thrombocytopenia
Topiramate (Topamax®)	Migraine headache	Yes	50 mg. qHS; daily max. dose 1500 mg	Kidney stone, glaucoma, weight loss
	Diabetic neuropathy	No		
Valproic acid (Depakote®)	Migraine headache	Yes	250 mg. bid; daily max. dose 500 mg	Rash can develop if used with lamotrigine
	Diabetic neuralgia, postherpetic neuralgia	No		
Zonisamide (Zonegran®)	Neuropathic pain	No	100 mg. per day; daily max dose 600 mg	Somnolence, Stevens-Johnson syndrome
Ziconotide (Prialt®)	Management of severe chronic neuropathic pain intolerant or refractory to other therapies	Yes	2.4–19.2 mcg/day via intrathecal infusion	Only used intrathecally; black box warning

References

1. Abdulla A, Adams N, Bone M, et al. Guidance on the management of pain in older people. Age Ageing. 2013;42(Suppl 1):i1–57.
2. van Ojik AL, Jansen PA, Brouwers JR, van Roon EN. Treatment of chronic pain in older people: evidence-based choice of strong-acting opioids. Drugs Aging. 2012;29(8):615–25.
3. McLachlan AJ, Bath S, Naganathan V, et al. Clinical pharmacology of analgesic medicines in older people: impact of frailty and cognitive impairment. Br J Clin Pharmacol. 2011;71(3):351–64.
4. Uppington J. Opioids. In: Ballantyne J, editor. The Massachusetts general hospital handbook of pain management. Third ed. Philadelphia, PA: Lippincott Williams & Wilkins; 2006. p. 104–26.
5. Brownstein MJ. A brief history of opiates, opioid peptides, and opioid receptors. Proc Natl Acad Sci U S A. 1993;90(12):5391–3.
6. Stanos S, Tyburski M. Minor and short-acting analgesics, including opioid combination products. In: Benzon H, Rathmell J, Wu C, Turk D, Argoff C, editors. Raj's practical management of pain. 4th ed: Elsevier, Mosby; 2008. p. 613–41.
7. Gasche Y, Daali Y, Fathi M, et al. Codeine intoxication associated with ultrarapid CYP2D6 metabolism. N Engl J Med. 2004;351(27):2827–31.
8. Prommer E. Levorphanol: the forgotten opioid. Support Care Cancer. 2007;15(3):259–64.
9. Franceschi M, Scarcelli C, Niro V, et al. Prevalence, clinical features and avoidability of adverse drug reactions as cause of admission to a geriatric unit: a prospective study of 1756 patients. Drug Saf. 2008;31(6):545–56.
10. American Geriatrics Society 2012 Beers Criteria Update Expert Panel. American geriatrics society updated beers criteria for potentially inappropriate medication use in older adults. J Am Geriatr Soc. 2012;60(4):616–31.
11. Hwang U, Platts-Mills TF. Acute pain management in older adults in the emergency department. Clin Geriatr Med. 2013;29(1):151–64.
12. American Geriatrics Society Panel on Pharmacological Management of Persistent Pain in Older Persons. Pharmacological management of persistent pain in older persons. J Am Geriatr Soc. 2009;57(8):1331–46.
13. Fine PG. Treatment guidelines for the pharmacological management of pain in older persons. Pain Med. 2012;13Suppl 2:S57–66.
14. Watkins PB, Kaplowitz N, Slattery JT, et al. Aminotransferase elevations in healthy adults receiving 4 grams of acetaminophen daily: a randomized controlled trial. JAMA. 2006;296(1):87–93.
15. Jefferies K. Treatment of neuropathic pain. Semin Neurol. 2010;30(4):425–32.
16. Skoglund LA, Skjelbred P, Fyllingen G. Analgesic efficacy of acetaminophen 1000 mg, acetaminophen 2000 mg, and the combination of acetaminophen 1000 mg and codeine phosphate 60 mg versus placebo in acute postoperative pain. Pharmacotherapy. 1991;11(5):364–9.

A Biopsychosocial Perspective on the Assessment and Treatment of Chronic Pain in Older Adults

Burel R. Goodin, Hailey W. Bulls, and Matthew Scott Herbert

Overview

Pain is commonly understood to be a normal sensation triggered in the nervous system as an alert to the possibility of injury and the need for rest and recuperation. In this instance, the experience of acute pain is adaptive and can be considered an expected consequence of illness, injury, or surgery, which most often resolves with healing. However, the experience of chronic pain is an entirely different matter. Pain signals keep firing in the nervous system for weeks, months, and even years beyond the expected period of healing or resolution of the source of pain. Often it is the case that the experience of chronic pain is not reliably associated with an underlying pathology or disease severity. Therefore, chronic pain does not appear to serve an instrumental role in protecting the sufferer or in otherwise promoting adaptation and adjustment.

Chronic pain is one of the most frequently reported and costly conditions in clinical settings, and it is often associated with substantial personal burden for those it afflicts. According to the Institute of Medicine's 2011 report, "Relieving Pain in America: A Blueprint for Transforming Prevention, Care, Education, and Research," over 100 million Americans suffer from chronic pain conditions [1]. This figure is greater than the number of individuals with diabetes, heart disease, stroke, and cancer combined. It has been conservatively estimated that the total annual costs of treating chronic pain range from $560 to $635 billion dollars, while the value of lost productivity due to chronic pain ranges from $299 to $335 billion [2]. Taken together, these data attest to the unfortunate reality that many Americans will suffer from chronic pain at some point in their lives, and the resultant economic burden of chronic pain and its treatment is of significant magnitude. Chronic pain continues to represent a formidable current and ongoing public health crisis.

B. R. Goodin (✉) · H. W. Bulls · M. S. Herbert
Department of Psychology, University of Alabama at Birmingham, Birmingham, AL, USA
e-mail: bgoodin1@uab.edu

Due to modern advances in environmental health (e.g., sanitation), preventive care, and medical treatments, the life expectancy of Americans has steadily increased over the past 100 years. As a result, a major shift in the age distribution of the American population is currently under way. In countries like the United States, it has been speculated that by the year 2050, the percentage of the population over 65 years old will rise from 17.5% to 36.3%, and the over-80 age segment will more than triple [3]. Unfortunately, advancing age is often accompanied by a corresponding increase in age-related diseases associated with painful sequelae, such as cardiovascular disorders, diabetes, cancer, osteoporosis, and degenerative joint disease. Chronic pain appears to disproportionately affect older adults, such that the prevalence of persistent pain climbs steadily with advancing age until at least the seventh decade of life. In community-based studies of non-cancer-related chronic pain, it has been shown that approximately 36% of adults in the United States aged 60–69 years report experiencing daily pain. That percentage was similar for adults aged 70–89 years but increased to approximately 56% for adults who were 90–99 years old [4]. Furthermore, estimated rates of chronic pain for institutionalized older adults range from 45% to 83% [5]. It is expected that as the US population ages and the risk of frailty and chronic diseases increases, the prevalence of chronic pain among older adults will continue to rise.

There is a growing clinical and research emphasis on chronic pain in aging populations. This is evident in the increased publication of empirical papers, the development of clinical guidelines and expert consensus statements, and the formation of special interest groups in professional societies such as the International Association for the Study of Pain as well as the American Pain Society [6]. Despite this increasing attention, chronic pain is frequently untreated or undertreated among older adults because of barriers in recognition, assessment, and management. For instance, a recent systematic review that examined the prevalence and treatment of pain among older adults residing in nursing homes revealed that approximately 40% of residents who reported pain did not receive any type of analgesic [7]. This review further demonstrated that acetaminophen was frequently administered as first-line therapy but often given on an "as-needed basis" at lower-than-recommended doses. Specific consequences of untreated or undertreated pain among older adults include anxiety, depression, social isolation, cognitive impairment, disturbed sleep, increased risk of falls, and decreased recreational activities as well as increased use of healthcare resources [8].

Given the limitations thus far in characterizing age-related pain patterns, it is not surprising that there are some common misconceptions about the pain experiences of older adult populations. Misconceptions regarding the chronic pain experiences of older adults can be perpetuated by clinicians and patients alike. One such errant belief often held is that pain is a common, unavoidable part of the aging process. If older adult patients believe this to be true, they may not seek appropriate pain relieving treatments. Similarly, if clinicians also believe that pain in older adults is unavoidable and untreatable, they may further reinforce this belief in their patients and subsequently offer suboptimal treatment or no treatment at all [6]. As a result, the patient may feel dismissed or embarrassed and decline to further advocate for pain treatment, effectively committing the rest of their life to be spent in pain. Other misconceptions about the pain experiences of older adults often include, but are not limited to, the following: (1) older adults are generally less pain sensitive than younger individuals despite conflicting reports, (2) older patients complain more than younger patients even though they supposedly experience less pain, and (3) common pain treatments such as opioid therapy are unsafe for older adult patients [6]. Difficulty communicating with certain older patients, such as those with moderate-to-severe dementia, can serve to reinforce these misconceptions in clinicians when the patient is unable to effectively self-report pain. Because of this, there is an ongoing movement to address and correct misunderstandings about the pain experiences of older adults and also improve pain assessment and treatment in aging populations [6]. Clinicians should strive to be aware of these common misconceptions and any resulting biases that unduly influence their pain assessment and treatment of older adults with chronic pain.

The primary purpose of this chapter is to provide a focused review of important topics related to pain assessment and treatment within a biopsychosocial framework that clinicians can apply toward better management of older adults with chronic pain. The assessment of pain in older adult populations should be comprehensive, involving evaluations of physical, psychological, cognitive, neuropsychological, and behavioral functioning [9]. A detailed general discussion of pain assessment is found in Chap. 2. Specific issues on chronic pain assessment are found here. It has been suggested that effective pain management in older patients should include both pharmacologic and nonpharmacologic strategies [8]. Pharmacologic strategies call for administration of non-opioid analgesics, opioid analgesics, and adjuvant medication. Polypharmacy, drug-drug and drug-disease interactions, age-associated changes in drug metabolism, and the high frequency of adverse drug reactions need to be carefully considered when the decision is made to use medications in this population [10]. Chapters 4 and 6 address specific unique physiologic considerations in pain management and recommendations for specific drugs, respectively. Nonpharmacological and complimentary interventions can also play a significant role in the management of chronic pain affecting older adults, including physical therapy, massage, low-impact physical activity, and electrotherapy, as well as cognitive-behavioral therapies and strategies to promote coping skills and increased functioning. This chapter addresses multiple modalities of pain treatment with particular emphasis placed upon the application of nonpharmacological and complimentary interventions to older adults' chronic pain.

Pain Assessment

Nociceptive and Neuropathic Pain

Chronic pain can be categorized along a variety of dimensions; however, arguably one of the most important divisions is nociceptive versus neuropathic pain. An initial step in the assessment of chronic pain in older adults is for clinicians to have an appropriate understanding of the differences between nociceptive and neuropathic pain. The differences can be very important for understanding the nature of the pain problem and especially for determining how to treat the pain.

Nociceptive pain is associated with the activation of nociceptors, or the nerve endings that transmit painful sensations. Common nociceptive syndromes in older adults are associated with joint or bone, muscle, skin, or connective tissue damage, either by trauma or degenerative disease [9]. Such conditions are often identified with visual inspection, X-ray, computed tomography, and magnetic resonance imaging. Superficial pains like those resulting from skin lesions or joint degeneration can be assessed with touch, pressure, stretch, and visual observation; they are often sharp, defined pains that are clearly localized. Deep tissue or visceral pains, on the other hand, can be described as dull aches and prove difficult to localize. Evaluating these deeper pains may require additional weight-bearing, mechanical, or active motion assessment [9]. Potential nociceptive disorders to evaluate specifically in older adults include osteoarthritis, low back pain, osteoporosis, myofascial pain, or regional pain disorders, among others.

Neuropathic pain is a type of pain that is associated with dysfunction or insult to the nervous system rather than the more typical peripheral nociceptor activation. As such, symptoms associated with neuropathic pain syndromes may be described differently in patient reports. Neuropathic pain sensations are often described as "shooting," "burning," or "tingling." Routine pain evaluation tactics are recommended for assessment of neuropathic pain, including perception of touch, vibration, cold, warm, pinprick, and position sense, with additional tests for neuropathy-specific aspects like allodynia, hyperalgesia, and hyperpathia [9]. Due to the complicated nature of diagnosing and localizing neuropathic pain, appropriate screening measures used are less obvious and poorly validated. Some suggested approaches have included nerve blocks, positron emission tomography and magnetic resonance imaging, and quantitative sensory testing methods, among others [9]. However, because these procedures can be both time intensive and financially consuming, they may not be reasonable assessments for brief clinical screenings. For more comprehensive information regarding the assessment of neuropathic pain, see the European Federation of Neurological Societies guidelines on neuropathic pain assessment [11].

For initial assessment purposes, awareness of disorders that are likely to involve neuropathic pain can be helpful, especially those most likely to occur in older populations. These disorders include herpes zoster, postherpetic neuralgia, central poststroke pain, trigeminal neuralgia, peripheral neuropathy caused by diabetes, HIV, and other related illnesses [9]. Additionally, the incidence of traumatic injuries such as falls may increase older adults' likelihood of spinal cord injury, which also often leaves neuropathic pain in its wake. Assessment of these conditions through interview, medical history, and self-report may be important in ascertaining the likely presence of neuropathic pain and determining the need for further neuropathic pain testing.

Functional Assessment

Chronic pain and aging are associated with impairments in basic physical functioning as well as the performance of activities of daily living (ADL). Older persons with chronic pain report more disability and ADL impairment than older adults who are pain free. Moreover, prospective studies of pain predict subsequent decreases in muscle strength and balance and increases in physical frailty, emotional distress, and activity avoidance [9]. Pain may magnify and accelerate age-related disability and functional decline, which, in turn, can increase the risk of falls for older adults. In addition, medications often used to treat chronic pain may heighten fall risks. For these reasons, mobility and balance should be routinely evaluated in older adult pain patients so as to assist with treatment planning (e.g., involvement of a physical therapist to optimize mobility and balance) [9]. The short physical performance battery (SPPB) is a well-validated procedure for objectively assessing balance and mobility [9]. The SPPB specifically evaluates lower extremity functioning based on timed measures of standing balance, walking speed, and ability to rise from a chair. The SPPB can be completed in 5 min or less by patients who are cognitively intact. Although this may still be too much time for some clinicians who may be restricted to 10–15 min per patient, a qualified assistant could complete the SPPB before the appointment.

In addition to the performance-based measures of physical functioning like the SPPB, there are also well-validated self-report measures of physical function that may be useful for the assessment of pain-related disability in older adults [9]. These measures should be considered an adjunct to clinical assessments and physical evaluations because the scope of the questions addressed by the instruments vary and may not be equally relevant to all older adult patients or chronic pain conditions. Many of the self-report physical function measures broadly evaluate patients' ability or difficulty in performing ADLs. ADLs are often categorized as either "basic," "instrumental," or "advanced" according to their degree of difficulty and the physical resources necessary for their successful completion. Basic ADLs include self-care (e.g., personal hygiene) and basic mobility. Instrumental ADLs are activities associated with independent living in the community (e.g., managing finances). The category of advanced ADLs was established to reflect activities that are discretionary and more physically and socially demanding (e.g., community involvement). Research suggests that it is advanced ADLs that are most likely to be impacted by chronic pain in older adults [9]. Examples of self-report functional assessment measures include the Physical Activity Scale (PAS) and the Pain Disability Index (PDI), both of which assess basic, instrumental, and advanced ADLs [9]. There are additional self-report measures of physical functioning that are well validated for the assessment of site-specific disability and take only minutes to complete. These include the Oswestry Disability Index (ODI; lower back) and the Western Ontario and McMaster Universities Osteoarthritis Index (WOMAC; hip and knee) among others [9].

Pain Assessment Tools

Self-Report Instruments

Self-report remains the "gold standard" of pain assessment. Despite obvious limitations in relying solely on patient report, no other approach has yet been able to overtake the patient's own account of their pain experiences. A variety of tools and approaches have been developed to record the self-report of older adults' pain, including specialized assessments for evaluation of neuropathic and cognitive impairment groups. Both verbal self-report via interview and pencil-and-paper measures can be helpful in ascertaining these aspects of the pain experience. An additional benefit of using self-report pain assessment measures is that they can easily be used to track the intensity and quality of pain over time, providing feedback on the effectiveness of treatment.

When conducting an initial pain interview, what the clinician wants to learn from self-report is the presence or absence of pain sensation, what factors may precipitate its onset, how often the pain is felt and where, the intensity of pain at any given time, and its ultimate impact on the patient's quality of life and independence. A formal pain interview is not necessarily required, but choices for these exist if structure is preferred. Any interview should strive to answer the abovementioned questions and also to explore pain using different terminology. Older adults may be reticent in reporting their pain if it is simply called "pain" but are sometimes more likely to respond to a variety of other terms like "bother," "ache," "sore," or "hurt" [9]. Conducting clinical interviews for pain assessment can even be effectively done with patients demonstrating some cognitive impairment, granted that these patients are still able to communicate in a lucid and coherent manner.

Older adults with intact cognitive abilities are typically able to give valid and reliable responses to most pain scales. Numeric rating scales (NRS), verbal descriptor scales (VDS), and specific measures like the short-form McGill Pain Questionnaire (SF-MPQ) or the Philadelphia Geriatric Center Pain Intensity Scale (PGC-PIS) are valid choices for evaluating pain intensity and quality throughout the adult life span [9]. An exception to this is the visual analog scale (VAS). Varying research exists, but some studies have shown that older adults have a more difficult time appropriately using the VAS than their younger counterparts [6]. Given the wide variety of pain assessment tools available, the VAS should be avoided in favor of other, more reliable measures.

Self-report measures have primarily been developed for nociceptive pain, but fewer validated measures exist for evaluating neuropathic pain. Examples of screener questionnaires include the Leeds Assessment of Neuropathic Symptoms and Signs (S-LANSS), Neuropathic Pain Questionnaire (NPQ), and Douleur Neuropathique 4 (more commonly known as simply the DN4). These measures have been shown to differentiate nociceptive and neuropathic pain, showing increases in responding for burning, cold, electric shock-like, shooting, and stimulus-evoked pain questions in the neuropathic group [9]. Additionally, two questionnaires can be used as a more comprehensive evaluation of the pain experience, the Neuropathic Pain Scale (NPS) and the Neuropathic Pain Symptom Inventory (NPSI). The caveat to these measures is that they have not been validated specifically in a large geriatric population, although they have been tested over the adult life span [9]. Given that these measures still need to be psychometrically validated with geriatric populations, they should be used with caution. However, the NPS and NPSI may still contribute useful information regarding the neuropathic pain experiences of older adults.

Noncommunicative Patients and Observation of Pain Behaviors

It is worth reiterating the importance of determining the ability of older patients to appropriately communicate with their clinicians and self-report their pain. Clinical interviews can be successfully used for some older adults with mild cognitive impairments. Further, even when cognitive impairments are suggestive of mild-to-moderate dementia, older patients may also still be able to reliably self-report their pain using VDS and NRS ratings if the instructions are repeatedly and carefully explained [6]. However, use of a VAS is still not recommended for these patients. For older adults with moderate-to-severe cognitive impairments and communication deficits, relying solely upon pain self-reports risks undermining the reliability of the pain assessment for these individuals. Accordingly, other informational sources should be sought out. For instance, clinicians are encouraged to become familiar with these patients' full health and pain history from records and family, attempt to observe their pain behaviors, and seek out other caregiver reports to ensure a comprehensive pain assessment is completed.

Research aimed at enhancing the overall quality of pain assessment, particularly for older adult patients, has identified a set of behavioral observations associated with having pain. These behaviors include such actions as guarding, grimacing, verbal or nonverbal expressions, rubbing, joint flexion, and bracing, among others. There are currently measures such as the Checklist of Nonverbal Pain Indicators (CNPI) or the Discomfort Scale (DS-DAT) that can be used by clinicians as brief tools to assist in the observation of pain behaviors [9]. In clinical practice, use of a single brief observational assessment of pain behaviors may make it difficult to appreciate the full range of pain behaviors often demonstrated by older adults. However, observing pain behaviors in conjunction with other ancillary sources of information (e.g., health and pain history) can provide greater insight into the location of pain as well as events that precede pain onset or exacerbate pain severity. Undoubtedly, behavioral observation can be helpful when assessing pain in noncommunicative older adults who may otherwise be unable to express their pain experience. Again, collaboration with an informant familiar with the patient (e.g., family member or caregiver) can be helpful for clarifying observational information.

It is important to note that the use of pain observation and brief observational tools among older adult patients with more advanced dementia should be done with caution. This is because the complex characteristics of dementia may affect the pain response in a variety of ways, such as psychomotor agitation or blunted behavioral responses. Brief assessment of a small number of pain behaviors risks minimizing the pain experiences of older demented patients and allowing false negatives to occur [9]. For this reason, extended observational measures have been developed for use with these individuals; one such example is the Pain Assessment Checklist for Seniors with Limited Ability to Communicate (PACSLAC). While no pain observation measure is without its psychometric shortcomings, the PACSLAC has preliminarily demonstrated excellent reliability and validity, and a review by pain nurses deemed this observational measure for demented older adults as "clinically useful" [9]. As such, the PACSLAC may be a worthwhile 5-minute observational measure to aid pain assessment in older adults with dementia. For more information regarding other brief and extended observational measures of pain, see the Expert Consensus Statement on Assessment of Pain in Older Adults [9]. Finally, while computer-assisted technologies to identify pain in elderly adults with dementia are currently being developed, further refinement and testing are needed prior to clinical use [12].

Psychological Functioning

Because pain is by definition a subjective phenomenon, it is closely intertwined with emotional and psychosocial processes across the life span. Psychosocial models of chronic pain development and perpetuation have become more prevalent in the literature; however, extension to populations of older adults remains limited. Psychosocial models of pain often include personality features, mood and emotions, as well as thoughts and beliefs pertaining to the pain experience. In laying out a comprehensive assessment strategy, it is important for the clinician to remember that these psychosocial domains can be closely related to the chronic pain experiences of older adults.

Personality

Stable personality traits can play an important role in the experience of pain and may moderate its long-term effects upon older adults' well-being. For instance, the personality feature of neuroticism (often characterized as a tendency toward anxiety, anger, envy, guilt, and depressed mood) is known to exert a strong negative influence on pain, perhaps through its effects on specific maladaptive cognitive and affective processes [9]. Conversely, dispositional optimism (characterized by positive expectations for the future) has been shown to predict less severe pain experiences and better psychological adjustment to chronic pain in older persons [13]. The NEO Personality Inventory is a straightforward, multidimensional measure that is appropriate for clinical use [9]. Given that the assessment of chronic pain in older adults is often restricted due to time limitations in the clinic, assessment of patients' personality features may best be completed in the context of a referral to a clinical psychologist as necessary. Clinical psychologists can usually spend more time conducting in-depth evaluations of pain patients' personality features and overall psychological functioning.

Mood and Emotional Responses

Chronic pain in older adults is often associated with increased psychological distress and mood disturbances. Key psychological constructs for consideration include depression and anxiety; in fact, depression and anxiety are extremely common responses to uncontrollable pain and are also frequently comorbid with other disorders of mood [9]. Further, anxiety and depression have a significant negative impact on performing ADLs in older adults, and therefore these conditions may warrant special attention [14]. It is important to note that a variety of behavioral manifestations can accompany depression and anxiety in chronic pain populations. These behaviors include sleep disruption, fatigue, disordered eating, and decreased physical functioning, all of which can result from the presence of chronic pain as well as exacerbate the experience of it. While these pain-related mood and behavioral disturbances are not necessarily specific to the elderly, older adults with chronic pain may experience symptoms of psychological distress in a different context than their younger counterparts. For example, older adults may find themselves coping with a variety of age-related issues such as fears of their own morbidity and mortality, changes in cognition, memory, communication, and/or physical functioning, relationship changes with family, grief from peer or family deaths, and loss of physical and financial independence. While some transient psychological distress and difficulty adjusting to the process of growing older can be expected, individuals with chronic pain have up to four times the incidence of mood disorders when compared to their pain-free counterparts. Therefore, psychological evaluation is an important part of older adults' pain assessment.

Because depression and anxiety are two of the most common psychological presentations affecting patients with chronic pain, several measures have been specifically designed for use with older adult populations. The Geriatric Depression Scale (GDS) is regarded as the standard for assessing depressive symptomatology and for preliminary screening of diagnosable depressive disorders in older adults. The GDS is well validated and simple enough to be used even for patients with mild to moderate cognitive impairments [9]. Alternatively, for patients with more severe cognitive impairments, the Cornell Scale for Depression in Dementia (CSDD) is well validated and easy to use. A reliable screening tool for anxiety is the State-Trait Anxiety Inventory (STAI), which can be used across the life span but has been specifically validated with older adults. The STAI provides insight into state (current) as well as trait (enduring) anxiety symptoms [9]. Other choices for general anxiety measures include the Beck Anxiety Inventory (BAI) and the Hospital Anxiety and Depression Scale (HADS), both of which are appropriate for use in cognitively intact older adults. Older adults have been found to underreport emotional symptoms, which could affect the validity of assessment conclusions [9]. As with the underreporting of pain, clinicians should be alert to this possibility and aim to overcome any barriers to reporting through the use of specific and pointed questions. However, if the patient is exhibiting clinically significant levels of depression and/or anxiety, a referral to a psychologist may be warranted to help minimize the severity of these symptoms.

Beliefs About Pain

Beliefs about pain are highly relevant for the assessment of pain in older adults. For example, if patients believe that pain is to be expected as part of normal aging and that it just needs to be tolerated, they may be less likely to report that pain to a clinical health provider. Along this line, there is growing evidence to suggest that stoic attitudes (i.e., attitudes demonstrating courage in the face of pain) are associated with the underreporting of pain in older adults living in nursing homes. Pain-related beliefs among older adults such as "if you have a pain, put up with it" and "what can't be cured must be endured" are indicative of stoic attitudes and have been found to be associated with lack of willingness to seek treatment for chronic pain [15]. Astute clinicians should be able to recognize such stoic beliefs and encourage older patients to report on their pain concerns without hesitation.

An important contributor to older adults' chronic pain experiences is the perceived ability (or lack thereof) to exert control over their pain. Patients who feel that they have no control over chronic pain are at high risk of psychological and functional impairment. It is important to consider that pain control beliefs often change with increasing age as a result of both maturation (i.e., learning what we can and cannot expect to control) and adaptation to changing abilities and circumstances. Among older adults who may be struggling with increasing loss of control and independence in other aspects of their life, such as a new transition to a nursing home, perceived inability to control their chronic pain may be particularly relevant. An important measure that clinicians should be aware of for the assessment of pain control beliefs is the Pain Locus of Control scale (PLC), which has been validated for use with older people [9, 15].

Perceived control over pain strongly influences choice of coping strategies patients engage when attempting to manage their pain. Patients who perceive little or no control over their pain more often engage in emotion-focused coping (vs. problem-focused coping) and passive coping strategies (vs. active), which have both been linked to poorer psychological adjustment in all age groups [9, 15]. Examples of emotion-focused and passive coping include venting about problems to others and ignoring the problem in the hope that it will go away, respectively. For older patients specifically, a common passive coping strategy is activity restriction and avoidance when confronted with pain. Activity restriction can lead to further social withdrawal, physical deconditioning, and social isolation [9]. Generally, patients who engage in emotion-focused and passive coping would be candidates for psychological intervention. The Chronic Pain Coping Inventory (CPCI) has been successfully implemented in older adults as a measure of coping strategies [9].

Special Consideration

Minority Aging

By 2050, 42% of the older adults in the United States are expected to belong to a minority ethnic group [3]. Thus, it is increasingly important to consider the ethnic background of patients when assessing for pain and disability in older adults. This is because experience of pain is often shaped by interactions among biological, psychological, and social variables, all of which can vary according to individuals' ethnicity. Some ethnic groups (such as African Americans) demonstrate a greater propensity to develop painful conditions that continue into older age, such as osteoarthritis, diabetic complications, or sickle cell anemia. Additionally, studies in the United States show that African Americans report greater pain severity, pain-related disability, and pain-related activity impairment than non-Hispanic whites [16]. Ethnic differences in pain experiences are not only found in the United States; for example, European studies have also shown that ethnic minorities report widespread pain more often than white Europeans [16].

Equally important to the discussion of ethnic differences in the prevalence and experience of pain is that ethnic minority patients have a heightened risk for undertreatment of pain by the healthcare system. While some of this risk has been attributed to ethnicity-related proxy variables such as lower socioeconomic status, the Institute of Medicine has suggested a variety of other factors to be aware of that may influence undertreatment of pain in minorities. These factors include stereotyping, healthcare provider bias, lack of clinical appropriateness of care, and persistent racial and ethnic discrimination [16]. Coupled with the previously discussed practitioner misconceptions regarding pain in aging populations, older minority patients stand an increased chance of poor assessment and subsequent undertreatment for their pain issues.

A final consideration for the assessment of pain in older ethnic minorities is the potential for differences in the pain treatment preferences of minority patients. Some studies have demonstrated that minority groups use complementary and alternative treatment methods at a higher rate than non-Hispanic whites [17]. Popular complementary and alternative medicine choices may include prayer, vitamins, exercise, meditation, and herbs, folklore, or additional traditional Eastern approaches, among others. While many complementary and alternative treatment approaches are often innocuous with minimal side-effect profiles when used on their own, there is the potential for harmful interactions when used in conjunction with conventional medicines and care. Alarmingly, the vast majority (up to an estimated 83%) of minority patients who use complementary and alternative treatment methods do not report it to their physicians.[17] Thus, clinicians should be aware of, and pointedly assess for, complementary and alternative treatments that older patients may be incorporating to self-treat their pain. Doing so will lead to better evaluation and understanding of minority patients' beliefs about pain treatment, expressions of their pain experience, and potential interactions between any conventional and complementary/alternative treatments.

Pain Treatment

Pharmacotherapy

Pharmacotherapy is an important component of treatment for older adults with chronic pain. However, the safe and effective use of medications is predicated upon clinicians' thorough understanding of the various patient-specific factors that can affect older adults' responses to pain-reducing drugs. For instance, other health comorbidities, drug-disease interactions, drug-drug interactions, treatment adherence, and cost are all important factors for clinicians to consider [10]. Age-related changes in drug metabolism attributed to reduced renal and hepatic function, higher fat-to-lean muscle ratio, and decreased serum protein levels can increase the risk of adverse reactions even when pain medications are administered at lower-than-recommended doses [4].

It has been suggested that the optimal pharmacological treatment regimen is one that not only has a good probability of reducing pain and associated disability but also improves function and quality of life [10]. The dosages of medications required for older adults to maximize their pain treatment outcomes are still a matter of ongoing debate. This is in part due to the fact that most pain-reducing medications have not undergone clinical trials in older cohorts and, therefore, do not have empirically derived recommendations for age-adjusted dosing. However, the generally accepted dosing adage is "start low and go slow," including low initial doses, slow up-titration, and lower maximal dosing [10]. The least invasive route of administration is also recommended [10]. Once a pharmacological treatment regimen has been started, clinicians need to establish realistic pain management goals with older patients to reach a level of comfort that can improve quality of life. Frequent monitoring and follow-up may be required to prevent adverse events such as sedation, falls, dizziness, gait disturbances, constipation, cognitive impairments, and respiratory depression [4].

Despite the safe and responsible prescription practices of clinicians, some older adults may not prefer or be able to tolerate pain medications for the treatment of their pain. It is in this context that the utility of nonpharmacological interventions becomes apparent. A number of studies have demonstrated the efficacy of nonpharmacological interventions in reducing pain intensity, pain-related interference, and pain-related distress across a variety of pain conditions [4, 10]. Furthermore, pharmacological therapy for chronic pain appears to be most effective when combined with nonpharmacological interventions [4, 10]. It is worth noting that interventional therapies (e.g., epidural steroid injections, spinal cord stimulation) represent another means of pain management for older adults that merits consideration; however, discussion of these modalities is beyond the scope of the current chapter. For additional information on the use of interventional therapies for older adults, readers can refer to Chap. 8 and to a recent review article addressing this topic by Abdulla and colleagues [5]. The remainder of this chapter is dedicated to the presentation of nonpharmacological interventions and complimentary therapies that can be applied to the management of pain in older populations.

Self-Regulatory Interventions

Due to the recognition of the important role that factors such as affect, cognition, behavior, and socialization play in the experience of pain, clinical scientists continue to develop interventions that positively affect these factors in an effort to alter the perception and experience of chronic pain. Designed specifically to assist patients with developing skills that make them more active participants in their own care, many early examples of these pain management interventions are collectively referred to as the self-regulatory approaches [8]. The theoretical underpinnings of these self-regulatory approaches demonstrate how biological and psychological factors interact to influence the perception of pain. Often referred to as the mind-body connection, the application of this conceptualization to chronic pain is such that chronic emotional and psychological unrest can contribute to the development and exacerbation of chronic physical pain, much like chronic physical pain can contribute to negative alterations in emotional, psychological, and physical well-being. Therefore, self-regulatory approaches utilize the mind-body connection by attempting to increase the ability to manage the symptoms, treatment, physical and psychosocial consequences, and lifestyle changes inherent in living with a chronic pain condition. Examples of self-regulatory approaches to chronic pain management include interventions such as biofeedback, relaxation training, and mindfulness [8]. The self-regulatory approaches, along with many other nonpharmacological and complimentary interventions, are often implemented by licensed health psychologists.

Biofeedback

Biofeedback training is a systematic methodology through which patients are provided with real-time feedback about a variety of physiological processes. The goal of biofeedback training is to develop an awareness of the circumstances under which these physiological processes change, so that patients can learn to voluntarily exert control over the bodily reactions associated with these processes. In the context of pain management, the physiological targets are typically factors that are directly associated with pain exacerbations or those related to emotional responses to the pain. Common biofeedback methods for treating pain include blood volume pulse feedback, electromyographic feedback, temperature feedback, galvanic skin response, respiratory, and encephalography feedback. Biofeedback training may be used as part of multidisciplinary pain management regimen and generally includes relaxation training. Previous research comparing older versus younger adults using biofeedback appears to show comparable results in both groups [5]. For example, older adults appear to readily acquire the physiological self-regulation skills taught in biofeedback-assisted relaxation training and achieve comparable decreases in pain as their younger counterparts [5].

Relaxation Training

Relaxation training is a self-regulatory approach that is often used in the context of biofeedback training and also as a component part of other psychological interventions (e.g., cognitive behavioral therapy). Relaxation training focuses on the identification of states of tension within the mind and body, followed by the application of systematic methods such as diaphragmatic breathing (deep breathing), progressive muscle relaxation, or visualization to reduce tension and to alter the perception of associated physical pain [8]. Pain is both a physical and emotional stressor; the resulting stress response often exacerbates the perception of pain by affecting physiological reactivity and mood (e.g., muscle tension or spasm, constriction of blood vessels, depressive symptoms). Relaxation training focuses on educating individuals about the relationships between stress and pain and seeks to empower individuals by teaching them systematic self-control methods for altering physical states (e.g., muscle tension) and psychological states (e.g., distress). Relaxation training has been shown to be effective for treating chronic pain conditions such as headache, osteoarthritis/rheumatoid arthritis, and low back pain in older adults [18].

Mindfulness-Based Therapy

One final and closely related self-regulatory approach for chronic pain management is mindfulness meditation. Rooted in the principles of Theravada Buddhism, mindfulness meditation is based on increasing intentional self-regulation of attention to what is happening in the moment. Mindfulness meditation is taught in the mindfulness-based stress reduction (MBSR) program developed at the University of Massachusetts Medical Center and is now offered in many academic centers across the country. Mindfulness techniques such as MBSR can be taught to older adults, and improvements have been noted on self-reported measures of pain and mood as well as physical functioning [18]. Similar in many ways to the previously described methods of relaxation training, the goals of mindfulness meditation include the attainment of both relaxation and greater focus of attention. However, mindfulness meditation emphasizes the attainment of stress reduction through increased moment-to-moment awareness of thoughts, sensations, and emotions as they arise, without reference to the past or future. In using this present-focused approach to pain management, one of the goals is to separate the sensation of pain from the thoughts that often occur in response to such sensations. These thoughts typically occur as a result of negative pain experiences from the past and project to the future, thus triggering emotional distress. By focusing attention only on the phenomenon of pain in the present moment, as if one is a detached observer, an individual can learn to separate the experience of pain from negative thoughts and resultant emotional distress that serve to make the pain worse.

Behavioral Interventions

The underlying premise for the use of behavioral methods in the treatment of chronic pain is that behaviors tend to increase in frequency when reinforced, whereas behaviors will often decrease in frequency when not reinforced or punished [8]. In the context of chronic pain, the behaviors that are targeted through behavioral strategies are often referred to as pain behaviors, which can include response patterns such as excessive verbalization of pain (grunting, sighing), frequent discussion about pain, facial expressions, guarded movements, or restriction of movement. These pain behaviors are commonly reinforced through social contingencies, such as responses from other people. Other people's responses can include expressions of sympathy, relieving the individual of responsibility for even basic activities of daily living (solicitousness), or verbal reinforcement of the individual's pain symptoms. The reinforcement provided by such responses serves to increase the pain behaviors and thus contribute to what has been referred to as the disuse syndrome in the context of chronic pain [8]. The disuse syndrome is marked by excessive pain behaviors that are in the service of decreasing physical activity, which may lead to physical deconditioning and increased risk for the development of worsening pain and other medical comorbidities (e.g., obesity). A major drawback to behavioral approaches for the management of chronic pain is the limited number of qualified clinicians (often clinical psychologists) who can implement such interventions. However, as discussed below, technological applications offer a promising way of reaching individuals (especially older adults) who cannot readily and repeatedly present to a healthcare center or who reside in areas with limited access.

Operant Behavioral Therapy

In an effort to reduce pain behaviors and avoid the resulting negative consequences (e.g., disuse syndrome), clinical psychologists have often applied operant behavioral therapy to the treatment of chronic pain. [8, 19] Pioneers of this therapy emphasized the need to reduce disability through the alteration of pain behaviors using methods to diminish the reinforcing nature of the responses to such behaviors and increasing the reinforcement of healthy behaviors. Thus, the model of operant behavioral therapy often involves close family members and friends who frequently are responsible for unknowingly contributing to the reinforcement of pain behaviors. Considerable empirical investigation has been conducted on the effectiveness of operant behavioral therapy for chronic pain, and strong empirical support for this method has come from both laboratory-based and clinically based studies of this treatment approach [19]. Elements of operant behavioral therapy have been incorporated into the broader treatment approach of cognitive-behavioral therapy (CBT) for pain, where cognitive elements are also addressed. Given the rise in popularity of CBT for chronic pain management, there are few examples in the recent literature in which operant behavioral therapy is evaluated in its pure form as a treatment for older adults. However, studies have shown that the use of operant behavioral therapy alone to incrementally increase activity level yielded improvements in disability and quality of life that were equal to those of more costly treatments [19].

Fear Avoidance

Another central concept in the field of behavioral pain management is fear avoidance. Based on behavioral principles, fear avoidance refers to the development of avoidant behaviors that are motivated by fear related to pain [8]. For some older adults, significant fear develops in the context of a painful condition. As a result, these individuals seek to avoid contact with the fear-provoking stimulus (pain) by engaging in behaviors that allow them to avoid the onset or exacerbation of pain (e.g., inactivity). This pattern of avoidance also contributes to the disuse syndrome described above. At the root of the fear-avoidance phenomenon are catastrophic thought patterns related to pain and its impact on quality of life. The pain-related fear is often tied to excessive worry about further injuring or reinjuring oneself if the choice is made to become physically active. This process has been termed kinesiophobia, implying that the efforts to avoid physical activity take on a phobic quality for many sufferers [8]. Recent advances in the treatment of fear avoidance have focused on the application of in vivo exposure techniques to assist the individual with systematically engaging in physical activities as a means of decreasing the fears that are strongly associated with such activity. Behavioral research has examined the utility of in vivo exposure to graded physical activity as a means of systematic desensitization for the reduction of fear avoidance. Results of this research showed significantly greater improvements on measures of fear of pain/movement, fear avoidance beliefs, pain-related anxiety, pain catastrophizing, and depression following in vivo exposure to graded physical activity [19]. The application of in vivo exposure to the treatment of chronic pain represents a significant advancement and one that potentially has merit for the chronic pain experiences of older adults. Clinicians, particularly psychologists, who regularly utilize behavioral treatments as part of their practice, are likely the best equipped for implementing in vivo exposure as a treatment for chronic pain in older adults.

Cognitive-Behavioral Interventions

Cognitive-Behavioral Therapy (CBT)

CBT is an empirically supported psychotherapeutic treatment that aims to help individuals resolve their problems concerning maladaptive emotions, behaviors, and cognitions through a goal-oriented, systematic procedure. Originally developed to better address the treatment needs of individuals with depression and anxiety disorders, over time CBT has been effectively applied as a treatment for a host of psychophysical disorders (e.g., insomnia, posttraumatic stress disorder, bulimia nervosa, and chronic fatigue syndrome), including chronic pain. The development of CBT for pain management originally contained primarily behavioral strategies, such as the aforementioned operant behavioral intervention. Over time, CBT evolved to include more cognitive aspects, such as the identification of negative automatic thoughts and replacement of these maladaptive thoughts with adaptive, beneficial ones. The cognitive aspects of CBT have been reviewed and found to contain critical aspects of treatment that not only reduce pain and increase functional ability but also stabilize mood and decrease disability. An important component of CBT for pain management is a treatment rationale that helps individuals with chronic pain to better understand that cognitions and behavior affect the pain experience, and CBT emphasizes the role that individuals can play in controlling their own pain. Another important aspect of CBT for chronic pain management pertains to coping skills training. Skills training may incorporate a wide variety of cognitive and behavioral pain-coping strategies. For instance, activity pacing and pleasant activity scheduling are used to help individuals maximize their functionality and quality of life. Training in distraction techniques such as pleasant imagery, counting methods, and use of a focal point helps individuals learn to divert attention away from severe pain episodes. Cognitive restructuring is used to help individuals identify and challenge overly negative pain-related thoughts and to replace these thoughts with more adaptive, coping thoughts. Throughout the course of a CBT treatment regimen, individuals are encouraged to apply their coping skills to a progressively wider range of daily situations. Individuals are taught problem-solving methods that enable them to analyze and develop plans for dealing with pain flares and other challenging situations. Self-monitoring and behavioral contracting methods are also used to prompt and reinforce frequent coping skills practice.

There is strong evidence that non-pharmacological interventions such as CBT are effective in decreasing chronic pain in adults and improving disability and mood [5]. However, few studies or clinical trials to date have focused on older adults. At this time, a limited evidence base suggests that older adult nursing home residents as well as community-dwelling older adults with chronic pain seem to benefit from CBT pain management interventions when offered individually or in a group setting [5]. Given the considerable evidence that individuals who receive CBT interventions demonstrate improved psychological and physical functioning, it appears that the use of CBT for older adults with chronic pain is worth clinical consideration.

Acceptance and Commitment Therapy (ACT)

ACT is a newer treatment approach within the family of cognitive behavioral interventions that is based on a unified model of human functioning, "psychological flexibility" or the ability to behave consistently with one's values even in the face of unwanted thoughts, feelings, and bodily sensations. Intervention according to the ACT model typically consists of three components: (a) awareness and nonjudgmental acceptance of all experiences, both negative and positive, (b) identification of valued life directions, and (c) appropriate action toward goals that support values. In its application to chronic pain, the ultimate goal of ACT is to increase the ability to fully contact the present moment and the psychological and physical content it contains in order to persist in or change behavior in the service of chosen life directions. ACT is similar to CBT in that it considers cognitions as an important variable that interacts with the pain experience but differs in its approach to cognitions. Specifically, ACT advocates for the nonjudgmental acceptance of thoughts as opposed to the restructuring of thoughts as advocated in CBT. Further, ACT asserts that pain and suffering are a normal part of the human experience and teaches clients how to manage this pain and suffering in order to pursue values-based activities.

ACT has been shown to be effective in improving physical and emotional functioning among adults with chronic pain [20]. Similar to CBT, there are a limited number of studies and clinical trials that have assessed ACT in older adults, although preliminary research suggest ACT is efficacious in older adults. Further, there is one study that showed older adults with chronic pain (age 65 and greater) were more likely to respond to ACT and younger adults with chronic pain (age 18–45 years old) were more likely to respond to CBT, suggesting ACT may be particularly well suited for older adults [21]. Additional studies are in order to confirm this finding.

Technological Applications of Cognitive-Behavioral Interventions

For many older adults suffering with chronic pain, it may be that cognitive-behavioral interventions are not available or access to this treatment modality is limited. One important barrier that might limit older adults' access to cognitive-behavioral interventions for chronic pain management includes the inability to independently access the metropolitan areas where the vast majority of healthcare centers offering multidisciplinary treatment for chronic pain (e.g., CBT) are located [8]. Unfamiliarity with the metropolitan area, confusion with navigating an academic medical campus, and financial barriers (e.g., parking fees) all represent formidable limitations for older adults when accessing specialty treatments such as CBT or ACT for chronic pain management. Therefore, obtaining access to quality pain care can be a challenge for many older adults. Such limited access and use of healthcare by older adults has compelled new research examining efforts to deliver treatments such as CBT and ACT where they reside rather than require these patients to travel to an urban healthcare center. For this purpose, Internet- and telephone-based intervention tools are being designed to meet the goal of increased access to healthcare for older adults in need of cognitive-behavioral interventions for chronic pain management. Preliminary evidence has shown that both the Internet and the telephone can be effective means for the delivery of variations of CBT [8] and ACT [22]. Further, ACT delivered via video-teleconferencing has been shown to be similar in effectiveness as face-to-face delivery [23]. Additional research is needed comparing these technologies with traditional face-to-face treatment. Regardless, Internet- and telephone-based cognitive-behavioral interventions provide noteworthy alternative pain management options for older adults that live in remote areas

Physical Activity and Exercise

Exercise

There is limited evidence that physical exercise benefits older adults living with chronic pain [5, 18]. These benefits include the alleviation of pain, improved psychological health, and increased functional independence, as well as improved postural and gait stability. While numerous studies support the benefits of physical exercise in various chronic pain conditions, this is not to say that physical exercise is indicated for every chronic pain patient. For example, physical exercise is not recommended for older adults with comorbid conditions such as uncontrolled arrhythmias, unstable angina, acute myocardial infarction, or congestive heart failure. When a patient is a suitable candidate for increased physical exercise, it is important to consult the appropriate clinician (physician, physical therapist) and tailor exercises to address impairments that contribute to functional problems (e.g., pain, limited range of motion, muscle weakness). For example, strengthening back and core muscles are indicated for patients with chronic low back pain, whereas strengthening the quadriceps is indicated for patients with knee OA. After identifying what exercises will be performed, it is important for the clinician to discuss the intensity (the amount of muscle exertion), volume (how long exercises will be formed), frequency (how often exercises will be performed), and progression (increasing intensity, volume, and/or frequency pending on the patient's response to the exercise program). In addition, it is important that the patient receive sufficient exercise education to not overly exert the body (e.g., reducing the intensity or avoiding exercises that cause acute pain, swelling, or fatigue). Indeed, properly educated older adults are more likely to modify their exercise program to suit their physical capacity and are more likely to adhere to a long-term exercise program.

Complimentary Therapies

Electrical Nerve Stimulation

Electrical nerve stimulation (ENS) has been used since the 1970s for the management of chronic musculoskeletal pain. The development of ENS was originally based on the gate-control theory of pain, which posited that counter-stimulation of nerve fibers produced by ENS reduces the perception of pain. There are two basic types of electrodes used for ENS: transcutaneous electrical nerve stimulation

(TENS) and percutaneous electrical nerve stimulation (PENS). Unlike the TENS unit, which does not penetrate the skin, the PENS unit consists of "acupuncture-like" needle probes that are placed in the soft tissue and/or muscle of an affected body site. It has been suggested that the use of TENS alone, or in combination with other pharmacological strategies, can be an effective approach to chronic pain management among older adults [5]. Age does not have a significant impact on reported TENS comfort. When combined with physical activity and exercise, PENS can reduce pain intensity and self-reported disability in community-dwelling older adults with low back pain [5]. It has been shown that these benefits can be maintained up to 3 months following a 6-week PENS intervention. In addition, ENS has been shown to improve physical activity, sense of well-being, and quality of sleep in adults (though not older adults) with various chronic pain conditions [5].

Massage

Massage therapy has a long history of demonstrating positive effects on musculoskeletal pain and chronic pain in general [24]. It is proposed that massage can increase serotonin and dopamine levels while enhancing the local blood flow as well as "closing the pain gate." Ten minutes of slow stroke back massage has been shown to reduce shoulder pain and anxiety in older adults with a stroke, and this effect continues for 3 days after the massage [5]. Older adults found this helped them to relax and sleep better. An alternative form of massage known as "tender touch" (gentle massage) does improve pain and anxiety among older adults with chronic pain living in a long-term care facility. Furthermore, this approach is said to improve communication among staff and residents [5].

Conclusion

Without a doubt, the management of chronic pain in older adults is a complex endeavor, which requires that attention be paid to biological, psychological, and social elements. An assessment and treatment approach that emphasizes these elements as contributors to the pain experience is often both necessary and desirable. Although pharmacological management is considered by many to be the gold standard for pain care, we highlight the growing literature describing efficacious non-pharmacological and complimentary interventions and emphasize their role as adjuncts to traditional pain management. In particular, self-regulatory interventions, cognitive-behavioral therapy, and complimentary therapies that include ENS and massage offer promise as effective adjuncts for a substantial percentage of older adults with chronic pain. Efforts should be made to integrate these treatments into research specifically aimed at older adult populations with the hope that 1 day they may become part of usual chronic pain care.

It is important that a word of caution be expressed at this point. Given the increasing number of lay providers of both non-pharmacological interventions and complimentary therapies for chronic pain management, we underscore the importance of adequacy as well as quality of training among those clinicians who administer these interventions. Although a reasonably large number of individuals receive training in interventional techniques such as CBT exercise prescription, for example (including clinical social workers, rehabilitation psychologists, and in some cases nursing staff), fewer individuals have adequate training to competently deliver these interventions in a manner that meets the needs of older adults. If any of the interventions or therapies mentioned in this chapter are deemed appropriate for an older adult patient with chronic pain, it is strongly recommended that it be provided by (or a referral made to) a clinician with adequate training and experience in this approach.

References

1. Committee on Advancing Pain Research, Care, and Institute of Medicine. Relieving pain in America: a blueprint for transforming prevention, care, education, and research. Washington, DC: National Academies Press; 2011.
2. Gaskin DL, Richard P. The economic costs of pain in the United States. J Pain. 2012;13:715–24.
3. Vincent G, Velkoff V. The next four decades: the older population in the United States 2010 to 2050. Washington, DC: US Census Bureau, US Government Printing Office; 2010.
4. Bruckenthal P, Reid MC, Reisner L. Special issues in the management of chronic pain in older adults. Pain Med. 2009;10(Suppl 2):S67–78.
5. Abdulla A, Adams N, Bone M, Elliott AM, Gaffin J, Jones D, Knaggs R, Martin D, Sampson L, Schofield P, British Geriatric Society. Guidance on the management of pain in older people. Age Ageing. 2013;42(Suppl 1):S1–S57.
6. Gagliese L. Pain and aging: the emergence of a new subfield of pain research. J Pain. 2009;10(4):343–53.
7. Takai Y, Yamamoto-Mitani N, Okamoto Y, Koyama K, Honda A. Literature review of pain prevalence among older residents of nursing homes. Pain Manag Nurs. 2010;11(4):209–23.
8. Kerns RD, Sellinger J, Goodin BR. Psychological treatment of pain. Annu Rev Clin Psychol. 2011;7:411–34.
9. Hadjistavropoulos T, Herr K, Turk DC, Fine PG, Dworkin RH, Helme R, Jackson K, Parmelee PA, Rudy TE, Lynn Beattie B, Chibnall JT, Craig KD, Ferrell B, Ferrell B, Fillingim RB, Gagliese L, Gallagher R, Gibson SJ, Harrison EL, Katz B, Keefe FJ, Lieber SJ, Lussier D, Schmader KE, Tait RC, Weiner DK, Williams J. An interdisciplinary expert consensus statement on assessment of pain in older persons. Clin J Pain. 2007;23(Suppl 1):S1–S43.
10. Christo PJ, Li S, Gibson SJ, Fine P, Hameed H. Effective treatments for pain in the older patient. Curr Pain Headache Rep. 2011;15:22–34.
11. Cruccu G, Anand P, Attal N, Garcia-Larrea L, Haanpää M, Jørum E, Serra J, Jensen TS. EFNS guidelines on neuropathic pain assessment. Eur J Neurol. 2004;11(3):153–62.
12. Hadjistavropoulos T, Herr K, Prkachin KM, Craig KD, Gibson SJ, Lukas A, Smith JH. Pain assessment in elderly adults with dementia. Lancet Neurol. 2014;13(12):1216–27.
13. Goodin BR, Bulls HW. Optimism and the experience of pain: benefits of seeing the glass as half full. Curr Pain Headache Rep. 2013;17(5):329–39.
14. Stamm TA, Pieber K, Crevenna R, Dorner TE. Impairment in the activities of daily living in older adults with and without osteoporosis, osteoarthritis and chronic back pain: a secondary analysis of population-based health survey data. BMC Musculoskelet Disord. 2016;17:139.
15. Herr KA, Garand L. Assessment and measurement of pain in older adults. Clin Geriatr Med. 2001;17(3):457–78.
16. Green CR, Anderson KO, Baker TA, Campbell LC, Decker S, Fillingim RB, Kalauokalani DA, Lasch KE, Myers C, Tait RC, Todd KH, Vallerand AH. The unequal burden of pain: confronting racial and ethnic disparities in pain. Pain Med. 2003;4(3):277–94.

17. Wardle J, Lui CW, Adams J. Complementary and alternative medicine in rural communities: current research and future directions. J Rural Health. 2012;28(1):101–12.
18. Morone NE, Greco CM. Mind-body interventions for chronic pain in older adults: a structured review. Pain Med. 2007;8(4):359–75.
19. Molton IR, Graham C, Stoelb BL, Jensen MP. Current psychological approaches to the management of chronic pain. Curr Opin Anaesthesiol. 2007;20(5):485–9.
20. Hughes LS, Clark J, Colclough JA, Dale E, McMillan D. Acceptance and Commitment Therapy (ACT) for chronic pain: a systematic review and meta-analyses. Clin J Pain. 2017;33(6):552–69.
21. Wetherell JL, Petkus AJ, Alonso-Fernandez M, Bower ES, Steiner AR, Afari N. Age moderates response to acceptance and commitment therapy vs. cognitive behavioral therapy for chronic pain. Int J Geriatr Psychiatry. 2016;31(3):302–8.
22. Buhrman M, Skoglund A, Husell J, Bergstrom K, Gordh T, Hursti T, Bendelin N, Furmark T, Andersson G. Guided internet-delivered acceptance and commitment therapy for chronic pain: a randomized controlled trial. Behav Res Ther. 2013;51(6):307–15.
23. Herbert MS, Afari N, Liu L, Heppner P, Rutledge T, Williams K, Eraly S, VanBuskirk K, Nguyen C, Bondi M, Atkinson JH, Golshan S, Wetherell JL. Telehealth versus in-person acceptance and commitment therapy for chronic pain: a randomized noninferiority trial. J Pain. 2017;18(2):200–11.
24. Reid MC, Papaleontiou M, Ong A, Breckman R, Wethington E, Pillemer K. Self-management strategies to reduce pain and improve function among older adults in community settings: a review of the evidence. Pain Med. 2008;9(4):409–24.

Interventional Strategies for Pain in Older Adults

Michael Bottros and Paul J. Christo

Overview

Pain management in older adults can be quite complex, as one must consider an older person's cognitive deficits, functional capacity, physical disability, fall risk, and organ function or dysfunction thereof. The most common method of pain control in the ever-increasing elderly population is pharmacotherapy as reported both by patients and their physicians. As a preponderance of patients is placed on multiple pharmacological agents including inflammatory, neuropathic, antidepressant, and opioid medications, the elderly are becoming subject to the complex interactions and risks associated with polypharmacy. Hence, the importance of interventional strategies in these individuals is increasingly being recognized as part of a multimodal approach to pain management. In his review, Ozyalcin proposed that when weak opioids have proven unsuccessful, therapeutic nerve blocks or low-risk neuroablative pain procedures should be employed to help reduce the need for, the medication intake of, and the side effects of stronger opioids [1]. Freedman also agreed that effective pain management in the elderly may be achieved through a multimodal approach with invasive techniques as well as medication and psychological therapy [2]. While there is controversy regarding the efficacy of interventional pain techniques, the quality of medical literature on the specific usefulness of these techniques in the elderly remains relatively poor.

M. Bottros (✉)
Department of Anesthesiology, Division of Pain Medicine, Washington University School of Medicine, St. Louis, MO, USA

P. J. Christo
Division of Pain Medicine, Department of Anesthesiology and Critical Care Medicine, The Johns Hopkins University School of Medicine, Baltimore, MD, USA

Epidural Steroid Injections

Lumbar Spinal Stenosis

Degenerative lumbar spinal stenosis (LSS) is a major cause of pain and a decrease in the quality of life in the elderly. It is a common condition that occurs in the aging spine of individuals greater than 50 years of age and incurs billions of dollars in healthcare costs each year [3]. The incidence of spinal stenosis in the United States is estimated to be 8–11% of the population, and as the "baby boomers" age, an estimated 2.4 million Americans will be affected by the disease by 2021 [4]. Spinal stenosis in older people is most commonly caused by degenerative lumbar disease leading to a narrowing of the vertebral canal, which may result in spinal nerve compression causing back or radicular pain, neurogenic claudication, and a limitation of walking distance. Spinal stenosis may be managed conservatively with physical therapy and/or analgesic pharmacotherapy. Surgery for spinal decompression is also an option and is generally indicated as an emergency in patients with intractable pain associated with numbness, weakness, or bowel/bladder incontinence. Treatment with epidural steroid injections (ESIs) has increased dramatically in seniors with varying degrees of success (Fig. 1) [5]. Friedly et al. reported an increase of 271% in lumbar ESIs from 1994 to 2009 in the Medicare population. While the use and cost of ESIs have escalated, there has not been a similar increase in evidence to support the long-term effectiveness of this treatment [6]. However, there is some evidence to support the use of spinal nerve blocks to reduce symptoms on a short-term basis [7].

In a prospective cohort study, Botwin et al. reported >50% reduction in pain scores in 75% of older patients (mean age 77 years) with unilateral radicular pain due to LSS using fluoroscopically guided transforaminal epidural steroid injections (Fig. 2) [8]. A limitation of the study was the small patient population and the need for a randomized double-blind trial. Tadokoro et al. treated 89 patients aged 70 years or older diagnosed with lumbar stenosis using in-hospital conservative therapy which included physical therapy and epidural steroid injections [9]. Approximately 35% of patients reported an improvement in subjective symptoms and 40.4% of patients reported no disturbance in their activities of daily living (ADL) at a mean follow-up of 57.2 +/− 4.8 months. In a recent randomized single-blind controlled trial in patients with lumbar spinal stenosis, Koc et al. found both epidural steroid injections and physical therapy to be effective in improving pain and functional parameters for up to 6 months [10]. While the mean ages of the treatment groups were ~60 years, a limitation of the study was the relatively low numbers included in each treatment arm. On the other hand, Shabat et al. reported failure of conservative treatment in LSS patients over 65 years old which included epidural or nerve root injections [11]. However, this was an uncontrolled study. Hence, there is some limited evidence to support epidural steroid injections for spinal stenosis in older patients.

Fig. 1 Fluoroscopic image of an interlaminar epidural steroid injection

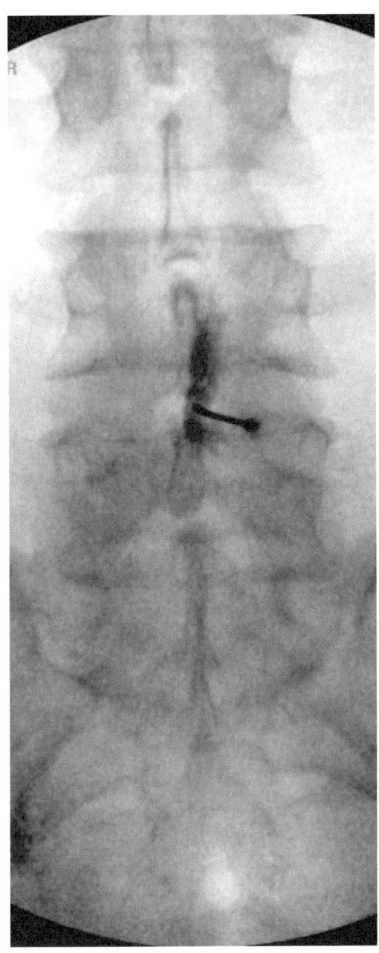

Sciatica

Sciatica is defined as "pain in the distribution of the sciatic nerve due to pathology of the nerve itself" [12]. This condition, which typically results from herniation of one or more lumbar intervertebral discs, has a lifetime incidence of 13–40%, is related to age, and peaks in the fifth decade [13]. Most patients who present with acute sciatica respond to conservative management over weeks to months [14]. In those that do not respond, surgery may be required, though in older people, surgery may be contraindicated or declined due to extensive comorbidities.

In the conservative model, sciatica is best approached from a multimodal, multidisciplinary perspective. However, epidural steroid injections have been used in its treatment for over 60 years with variable success [15]. While there

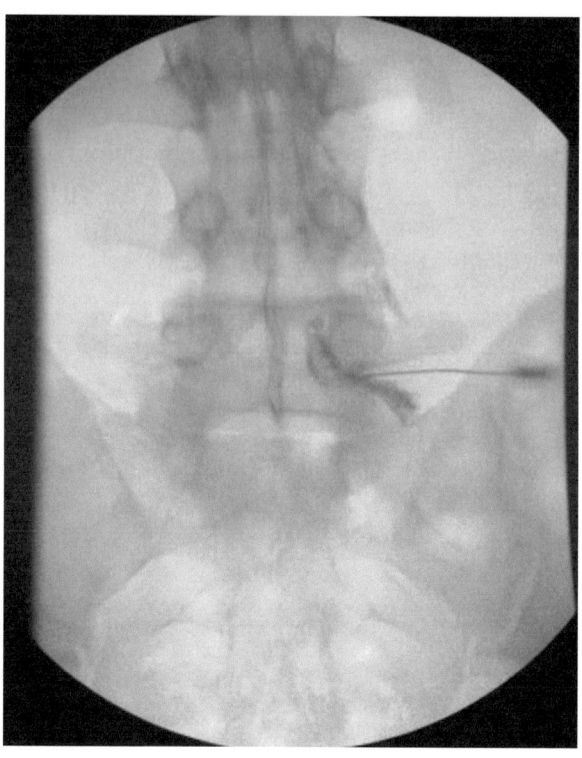

Fig. 2 Fluoroscopic image of a transforaminal epidural steroid injection

are no studies specific to the elderly population, most studies include all age groups. In a meta-analysis on efficacy of epidural steroids for sciatica, Watts et al. showed that the odds ratio for short-term benefit (up to 60 days) was 2.61 (95% CI1.9–3.77) and for long-term benefit, 1.87 (95% CI: 1.31–2.68) for epidural steroid compared with placebo [16]. This was independent of the caudal or interlaminar route of administration. The number needed to treat (NNT) for short-term benefit of >75% pain relief was 7.3. For >50% pain relief, the NNT was 3. Studies looking at long-term benefit of 12 weeks to 1 year report an NNT for 50% pain relief of 13 [17]. In a systematic review by Abdi et al., of the 11 randomized trials included in the evaluation of sciatica, 7 were positive for short-term relief (<6 weeks), whereas only 2 studies were positive for long-term relief (>6 weeks).

In a well-designed, prospective, randomized, controlled, double-blind study, Riew et al. demonstrated that transforaminal epidural steroid injections were significantly more effective than local anesthetic injections alone and decreased the need for surgical decompression for up to 13–28 months following injections [18]. In the most recent review of epidural injections for spinal pain, Bicket et al. included 43 studies totaling 3641 patients indirectly comparing epidural steroid, epidural nonsteroid, and nonepidural injections [19]. The study suggested that epidural nonsteroid injections were more likely than nonepidural injections to achieve positive outcomes (risk ratio, 2.17; 95% CI, 1.87–2.53) and provide greater pain score reduction (mean difference, −0.15; 95% CI, −0.55 to 0.25). They concluded that epidural nonsteroid injections may provide improved benefit compared with nonepidural injections on short-term (less than or equal to 12 weeks) outcomes.

In conclusion, there is some limited evidence to support epidural injections (steroid or nonsteroid) for radicular pain or sciatica.

Facet Joint Injections and Radiofrequency Ablation

The lumbar facet joints are true synovial joints with a fibrous capsule surrounding an articular surface and a synovial membrane, located at the junction of the superior articular process of the caudal vertebra and the inferior articular process of the cephalad vertebra (Fig. 3) [6]. While low back pain is a common complaint in older people, the typical features of facet-mediated pain include unilateral or bilateral low back pain, frequently referred to the buttock, hips, or thighs but infrequently below the knees. Facet "loading" refers to the exacerbation of pain by twisting or extension of the back which is sometimes relieved by forward flexion, rest, or walking. This was first described in 1988 from a small (22 patients) retrospective study of facet injections [20], but facet loading has not been found to be predictive of outcomes in larger studies [21]. It appears that paraspinous muscle tenderness may be the one physical examination feature associated with positive facet outcomes. Facet arthrosis and osteoarthritis are common radiological findings, and controlled studies of chronic low back pain have revealed a prevalence of facet joint involvement in 15–45% of cases [22]. The prevalence appears to be greater as one ages: Manchikanti et al. found the prevalence of lumbar facet joint-mediated pain confirmed by diagnostic nerve blocks to be 52% in the elderly, compared with 30% in all adults [23]. This pattern does not appear to hold true in chronic neck pain. In a retrospective analysis of 424 patients undergoing comparative nerve blocks, Manchikanti et al. showed that facet joint involvement in cervical pain was similar across all age groups [24].

From an interventional perspective, facet joint-mediated pain may be managed with intra-articular (IA) injections, medial branch nerve blocks, or radiofrequency ablation (RFA or denervation) (Fig. 4) of the medial branch nerves. The effectiveness of IA facet joint injections remains controversial. Most systematic reviews have concluded that injecting steroids into facet joints is ineffective [21]. At best, it provides only immediate-term relief in only a proportion of people with an inflammatory component and is less frequently favored than medial branch nerve blocks [25]. Medial branch nerve blocks are considered the best approach in the identification of a painful facet joint and serve as a more diagnostic or rather "prognostic" injection to predict outcome of denervation treatment. As Cohen et al. state, "Obtaining prolonged benefit from anaesthetic blockage of the nerves that innervate the facet joints is analogous to treating osteoarthritis by block pain signal transmission, and runs counter to the rationale behind comparative diagnostic blocks." [21] Should individuals obtain >50–80% relief from medial branch nerve blocks, patients

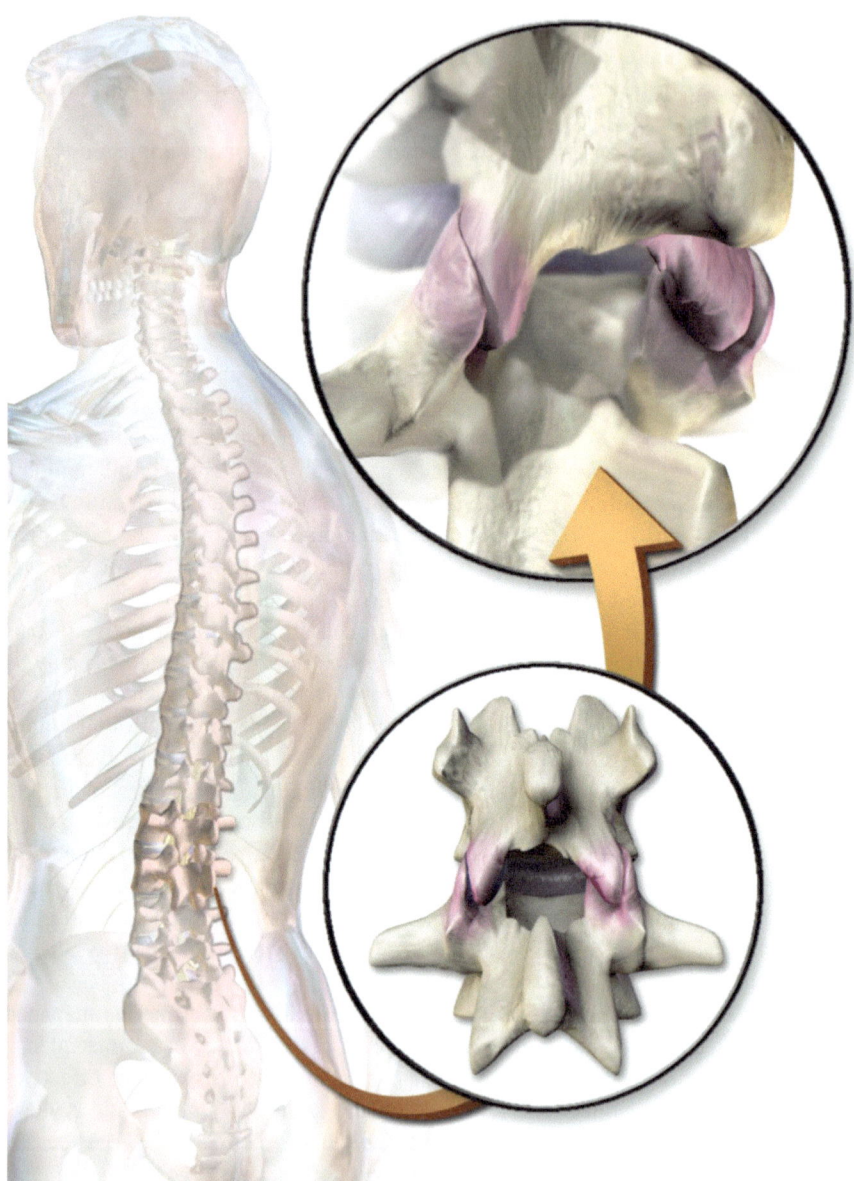

Fig. 3 Facet joint of the level of L4–L5. Blausen.com staff (2014). "Medical gallery of Blausen Medical 2014". WikiJournal of Medicine 1 (2). https://doi.org/10.15347/wjm/2014.010. ISSN 2002-4436. - Own work

progress to RFA which inactivates the afferent nerve supply to the joint for a period of time, typically 6 months to 1 year.

The evidence for radiofrequency denervation of the medial branch nerves, although mixed, is more supportive. A recent review of radiofrequency treatment of the ramus medialis of the lumbar ramus dorsalis (facet denervation) looked at seven

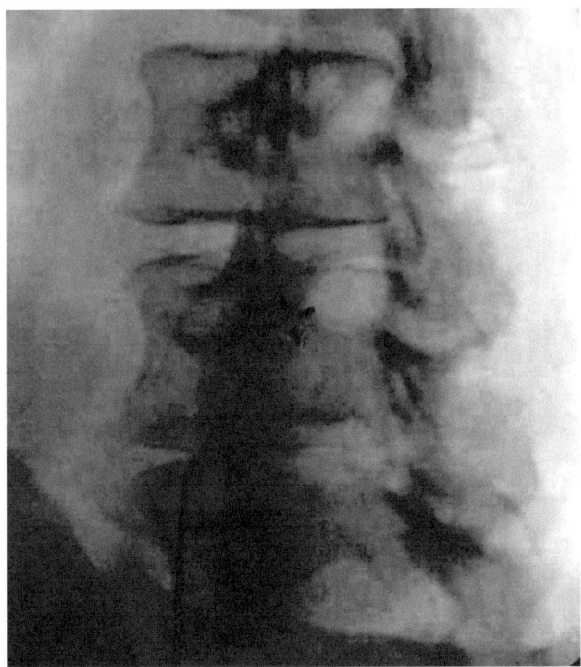

Fig. 4 Fluoroscopic image of a radiofrequency denervation cannula at the level of L4–L5

randomized controlled trials of which five were positive, one was equivocal, and one was negative [26]. The correct diagnosis of the condition is considered paramount, with rigorous pre-assessment of diagnostic facet nerve blocks. For example, in a study published by van Kleef, 31 patients out of 100 were included after a 1-h assessment post-diagnostic medial branch blocks with a reported prevalence of 31% for facet pain [27]. The number needed to treat was 1.6 in this study as compared to 11 when intra-articular facet injections were performed and assessed by a family doctor 24 h later [28]. van Eerd et al. reviewed the evidence for the treatment of cervical facet pain and concluded that radiofrequency treatment of the medial branch nerve could be considered for degenerative facet joint pain [29]. False positive rates have been reported from 15% to 40% and may be due to placebo response or spread of the local anesthetic. Serious complications and side effects are rare and are either related to the injectate or improper needle position [30]. All authors have highlighted the need for further randomized controlled studies.

In conclusion, the evidence in all age groups for facet joint interventions is mixed, although it is more supportive for RFA of the medial branch nerves.

Sacroiliac Joint Interventions

The sacroiliac (SI) joint is a diarthrodial joint that can rotate in all three axes and is designed primarily for stability (Fig. 5). It is the largest axial joint in the body, with an average surface area of 17.5 cm^2 [31, 32]. The SI joint may begin to display degenerative changes as early as puberty, progressing to painful symptoms in the

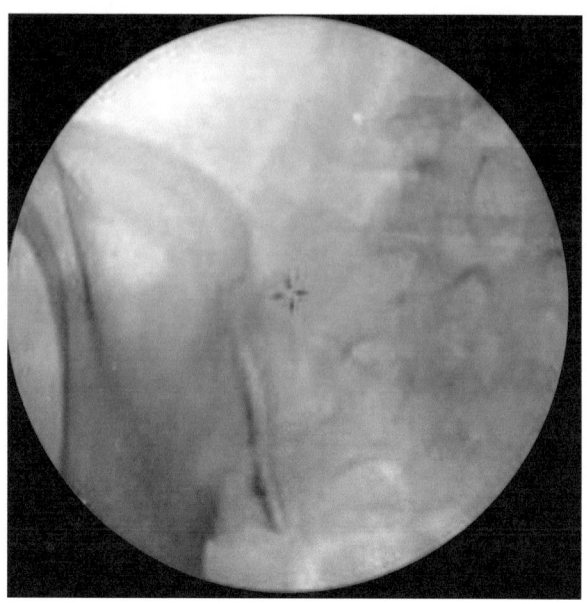

Fig. 5 Fluoroscopic image of the left sacroiliac joint

sixth decade of life when there is peri-capsular ankylosis. By the eighth decade of life, marked erosion and plaque formation are ubiquitous [33]. The sacroiliac joint accounts for approximately 16–30% of cases of chronic mechanical low back pain [34]. The most common referral patterns for SI-mediated low back pain can be the buttock (94%), lower lumbar region (72%), lower extremity (50%), groin (14%), upper lumbar region (6%), and abdomen (2%) [35]. Physical examination and radiographic imaging offer less sensitivity and specificity than small-volume local anesthetic diagnostic blocks [36]. Thus these blocks have become the "gold standard" of diagnosing SI joint pain [37].

Interventions for SI joint pain include proliferative therapy (prolotherapy), intra- (IA) and extra-articular (EA) injections of steroids with local anesthetics, and RF denervation [36]. Prolotherapy involves injecting nonpharmacological irritant solutions around tendons or ligaments to strengthen connective tissue and relieve musculoskeletal pain. The hypothesis is that by initiating an inflammatory process, there will be an enhancement in blood flow and thus an acceleration in tissue repair. Kim et al. compared IA 25% dextrose injections to steroid injections in the only randomized study regarding prolotherapy for SI joint pain [38]. Both groups had significant improvement at 2-week follow-up, though at 15 months, 58.7% of patients who received prolotherapy continued to experience a positive outcome versus 10.2% in the IA steroid group. However, due to the absence of placebo-controlled studies, one cannot recommend prolotherapy at this time.

Two controlled trials evaluated EA injections, both showing significant improvement in the treatment group at 1- and 2-month follow-up [39, 40]. IA injection of LA and steroid has been shown in various studies to be both diagnostic and therapeutic for a duration of 6 months to 1 year [36]. In his recent systematic review,

Rupert et al. demonstrated level II-2 evidence for diagnostic SI joint injections, level III-3 for RF neurotomy, and no evidence supporting or refuting therapeutic intra-articular SI joint injections [41]. In conclusion, the current literature supports the use of diagnostic SI joint injections followed by therapeutic RF neurotomy SI-mediated low back pain.

Vertebral Augmentation: Vertebroplasty and Balloon Kyphoplasty

Each year, worldwide, there are approximately 1.4 million vertebral compression fractures that present for pain or instability [42]. Osteoporosis is a common cause of these fractures, and the resulting acute pain may persist for weeks or months, even after the fracture has healed. The incidence of compression fractures in women >50 years of age is about 26% and increases to 40% at 80 years of age or greater [43, 6]. Pain symptoms are present in up to 84% of vertebral compression fracture cases, as well as pulmonary dysfunction, immobility, spinal deformity, chronic pain, and depression [44].

While the gold standard has been conservative medical management, vertebral augmentation via two procedures, namely, vertebroplasty (VP) and kyphoplasty (KP), has been advocated as the preferred treatment for painful osteoporotic vertebral fractures [45]. Both VP and KP involve minimally invasive surgery. VP consists of a percutaneously placed needle into the fractured vertebral body (either via an intra-pedicular or extra-pedicular approach) under imaging (Fig. 6) and injection of an acrylic cement called polymethyl methacrylate (PMMA) (Fig. 7). It was originally developed to treat vertebral angiomas [46] though it has expanded to include vertebral fractures from multiple myeloma, cancer metastases, avascular necrosis,

Fig. 6 Needle placement for vertebroplasty under fluoroscopy

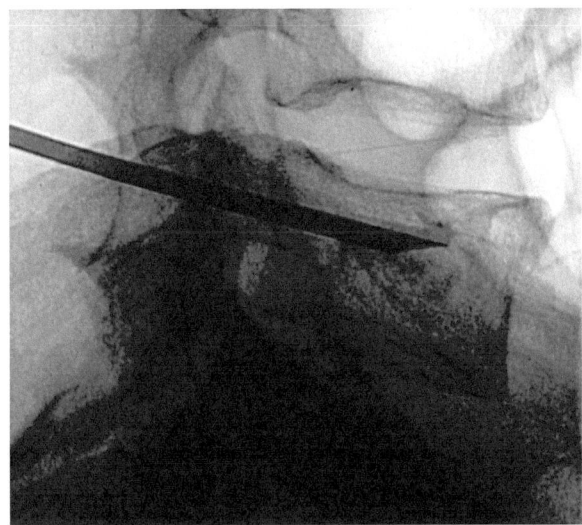

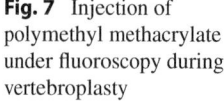

Fig. 7 Injection of polymethyl methacrylate under fluoroscopy during vertebroplasty

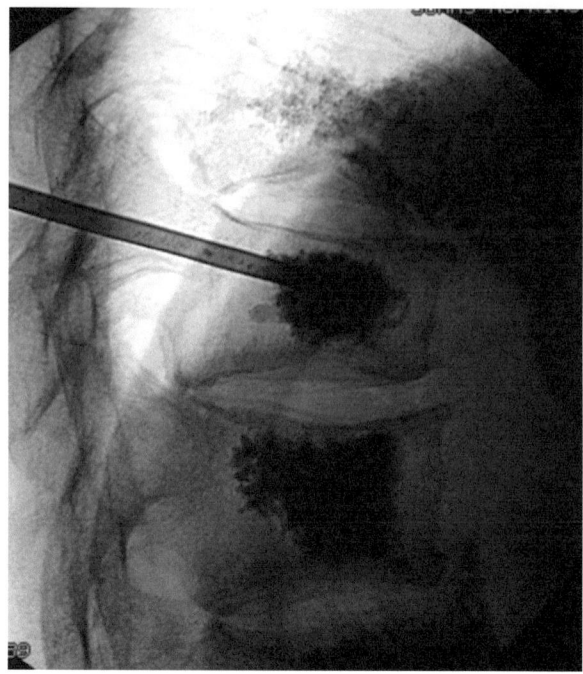

and osteoporosis as well. Kyphoplasty involves the inflation of a percutaneously delivered balloon in the vertebral body via imaging before injection of PMMA into the cavity created by the balloon (Fig. 8). KP offers the advantage of partial restoration of vertebral height and correction of angular deformity by this balloon inflation [22]. Single- or multiple-level VP may be done in one session [47].

Not all patients are amenable to VP or KP. Absolute contraindications include bleeding disorders, unstable fracture due to posterior element involvement, and a lack of a definable level of vertebral collapse. Relative contraindications are patient's inability to lie prone for the expected procedure duration (1–2 h), lack of surgical backup or patient monitoring facilities, and the presence of neurological signs and symptoms caused by vertebral body collapse or tumor extension (Table 1) [48]. VP and KP have a reported complication rate of 5% including bleeding, infection, rib or pedicle fracture, neurologic injury (root pain and radiculopathy), or cement leakage [49]. Serious complications include neuropathy or paraplegia resulting from cement extravasation into the spinal canal [50] or systemic extravasation of cement leading to pulmonary embolism in 3.5–23% of VP (though reportedly lower in KP) cases [51].

Several randomized and non-randomized clinical trials as well as case series have shown the immediate substantial reduction in visual analogue scores (VAS), improved functional status, and short-term efficacy of VP and KP [47, 48, 52–54]. The majority of patients in the reported studies were women aged 60 years and over. Significant pain relief is noted within 24 h after the procedure, and most are able to leave the hospital on the same day or following an overnight stay. The need for

Fig. 8 Kyphoplasty

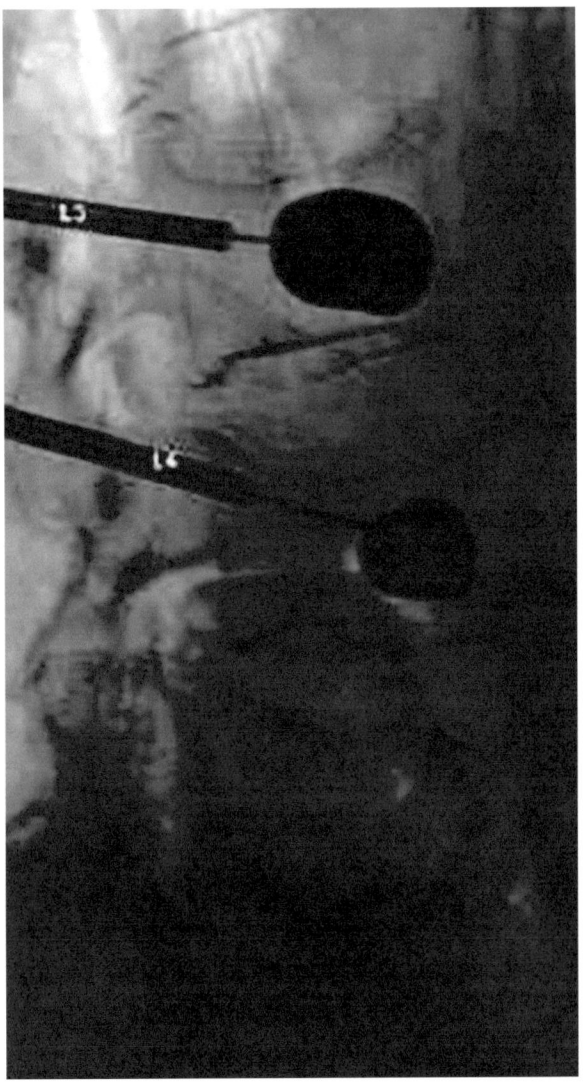

narcotic analgesics was also shown to be reduced for 6 months to 1 year [55]. In the first prospective randomized study supporting the efficacy and safety of VP in patients with acute compression fractures, the VERTOS II (Percutaneous Vertebroplasty Versus Conservative Therapy) study compared VP to conservative management for acute osteoporotic compression fractures in an open-label randomized trial [56]. In that study, 202 patients over the age of 50 years (mean age, 75 years) with acute compression fractures were randomized to either VP or conservative treatment and followed up at 1-month and 1-year intervals. Those who underwent VP reported a statistically significant reduction in VAS scores compared to the conservative treatment group. The difference between groups in reduction of mean

Table 1 Contraindications to vertebral augmentation

Absolute contraindications
Patient refusal
Bleeding disorders
Unstable fracture due to posterior element involvement
Lack of a definable level of vertebral collapse
Relative contraindications
Inability to lie prone
Lack of surgical backup or patient monitoring facilities
Presence of neurological signs and symptoms caused by vertebral body collapse or tumor extension

VAS score from baseline was 2.6 (95% CI, 1.74–3.37) at 1 month and 2.0 (95% CI, 1.13–2.80) at 1 year.

Similar results have been reported with KP. In a randomized controlled trial that included 300 patients, Wardlaw et al. showed that KP was associated with greater improvement in back pain, physical function, mobility, and quality of life than conventional medical treatment for at least 6–12 months [57]. The differences between the KP and medical treatment groups diminished after 12 months. However, in a 2-year follow-up study, Boonen et al. showed greater improvement in back pain over 24 months for kyphoplasty (overall treatment effect −1.49 points, 95% CI −1.88 to −1.10); the difference between the groups remained statistically significant at all time points at 24 months (−0.80 points, 95% CI −1.39 to −0.20) [58].

Two controversial trials challenged the reported benefits of VP [59, 60]. Both were blinded randomized controlled trials with sham surgery as the control comparator rather than conventional medical treatment. There was a noted improvement in VAS pain scores in both VP and control "sham-treated" groups in both studies, but no significant benefit of VP was found at 1-week and 1-, 3-, and 6-month intervals compared with the control group. However, several notable concerns have been raised regarding these trials. The studies defined fracture acuity by different standards than elsewhere in the VP literature, namely, that an "acute" fracture was defined as less than 1 year old, whereas an acute fracture is typically considered less than 4–6 weeks old. The control group in both trials underwent infiltration of the facet joint or periosteum with local anesthetic, which may have contributed to the placebo effect of injection and/or local anesthetic on its own as being effective. Also, pain outcomes may have been biased by an apparent lack of effort to determine whether the patient's pain was attributable to the compression fracture or something else. It is important to note that the degree of pain reduction in the VP groups was similar in these two trials and consistent with the benefits reported in previous uncontrolled and controlled trials [22].

Anderson et al. reported a recent meta-analysis of vertebral augmentation compared with conservative treatment for osteoporotic spinal fractures [61]. The authors showed greater pain relief, functional recovery, and health-related quality of life with cement augmentation compared with controls. Cement augmentation results were significant in the early (<12 weeks) and late time points (6–12 months). This meta-analysis provides strong evidence in favor of cement augmentation in the treatment of symptomatic compression fractures.

There has been long-standing debate over the superiority and safety of VP vs KP. Data from eight studies with 848 patients were extracted showing that in the first week, VP was superior to KP, at 3 months KP was better than VP, and at 1-year there was no difference in functional improvement and pain relief between the two groups [62].

In conclusion, while more randomized controlled trials are needed for a conclusive statement, there is good evidence from level I studies that support the use of VP for osteoporotic compression fractures and fair evidence for KP from level II and III studies. Intervention within the first 7 weeks of the compression fracture yields greater pain reduction than those treated later.

Neuromodulation

Neuromodulation is the precise delivery of electrical current or drugs to the nervous system. The concept has evolved to encompass both disease states that cause pain as well as other end-organ dysfunction, such as bowel/bladder dysfunction, peripheral vascular disease, and arrhythmia. The first successful use of neuromodulation for pain was in 1967 by Norman Shealy, a neurosurgeon in La Crosse, Wisconsin [63], using spinal cord stimulation (SCS). For the purposes of this section, we will limit discussion of neuromodulation to that of SCS.

Spinal cord stimulation involves the placement of a lead over a neural target in the spine via epidural placement (Fig. 9). Spinal cord stimulation has been used for over 35 years to help treat various pain states. It is currently approved by the US Food and Drug Administration (FDA) to aid in the management of difficult-to-treat chronic pain of the body and limbs, failed back surgery syndrome (FBSS), low back pain, and leg pain. Table 2 reviews the chance of success based on disease state. The procedure involves delivering a pulsed electrical field to the dorsal columns of the spinal cord from an electrical generator, supplied by an implanted battery or external radiofrequency transmitter. By using a programmable generator, the amplitude, rate, frequency, and shape of the electrical field can be manipulated to create pain relief.

Although the exact mechanism of action is unclear, spinal cord stimulation may be partly explained by the gate control theory of pain advanced by Wall and Melzack [64]. The mechanism of neural effect has been theorized to change the balance of inhibitory to excitatory fiber activity by the gate control process, by manipulating the number and position of cathodes and anodes on the lead [65].

In the past, SCS was considered mostly a last resort for those that have failed other conservative measures; however recent advances have changed this notion. SCS trials have been greatly simplified and are mostly done percutaneously as outpatient procedures (Fig. 10) guided by fluoroscopy (Fig. 11). After successful trial, electrodes are implanted into the dorsal epidural space percutaneously or by laminectomy. Mekhail et al. showed a substantial cost savings for patients undergoing

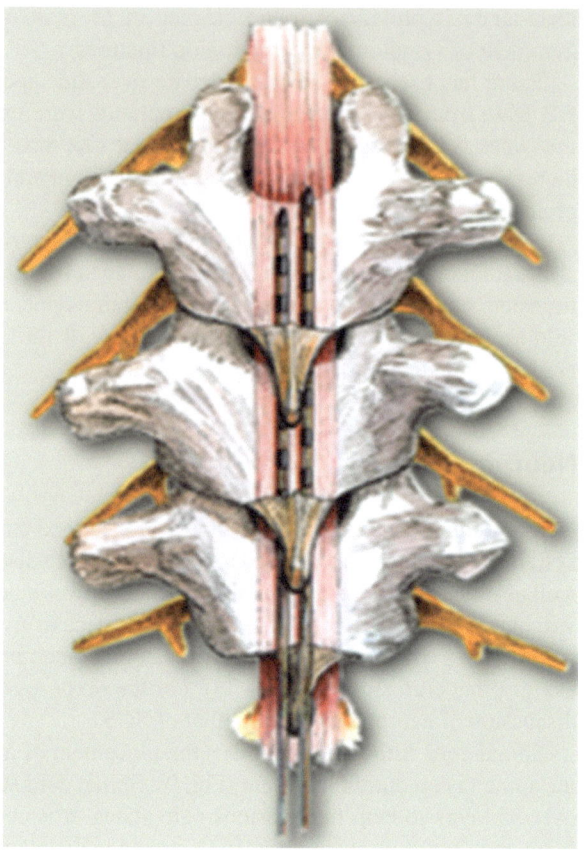

Fig. 9 Placement of percutaneous lead along the dorsal column of the spinal cord

SCS for neuropathic pain as compared to other treatment options [66]. Several randomized trials have shown positive long-term benefits in pain control with SCS. North et al. conducted a randomized controlled trial of 50 patients who either underwent SCS or reoperation for the treatment of FBSS [67]. SCS was found to be more effective than reoperation at 3-year follow-up with a reduced need for opiate analgesics in the SCS group as well as significantly fewer patient crossovers from the SCS group to the surgical group. Kumar et al. compared SCS plus medical therapy to medical treatment alone in 100 patients with FBSS. They showed that stimulation was superior to conventional medical treatment alone in that patient population [68]. Approximately 48% of patients undergoing SCS vs 9% of patients with medical management reached the primary outcome of 50% or greater pain relief at the 1-year follow-up. Complications from SCS therapy include electrode migration (10%), wound infection (8%), and loss of paresthesia (7%).

While no studies of SCS are specific to the elderly, the increasing body of evidence suggests that stimulation should be considered much earlier in the treatment algorithm for diseases causing neuropathic pain. SCS should be considered prior to a second back surgery in those without impending neurological compromise before chronic long-term opioids in those with neuropathic pain.

Table 2 Probability of successful pain reduction by SCS

High probability
Chronic cervical or lumbar radicular pain syndromes
CRPS I and II
Painful peripheral mononeuropathies
Angina pectoris – refractory to conventional drug therapy and not surgical bypass candidate
Painful ischemic PVD – refractory to conventional drug therapy and not surgical bypass candidate
Moderate probability
Axial low back pain
Pelvic pain
Postherpetic neuralgia
Visceral pain syndromes of the abdomen
Low probability
Neuropathic pain following spinal cord or brain injury
Nerve root avulsion, stretching or injury
Nerve root destruction after intentional iatrogenic procedures
Phantom limb pain

CRPS complex regional pain syndrome, *PVD* peripheral vascular disease
Adapted from Deer and Masone [65]

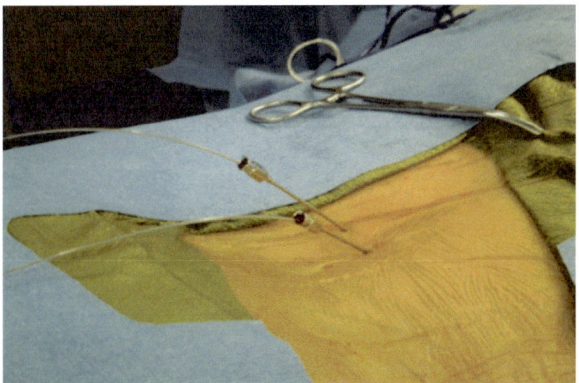

Fig. 10 Outpatient percutaneous SCS lead placement

Continuous Intrathecal Analgesia

Since the discovery of central opioid receptors in the 1970s, neuraxial infusions have been used in the treatment of both malignant and nonmalignant pain, by delivering certain analgesics to regions of the dorsal horn of the spinal cord, namely, lamina II (Fig. 12) [69]. No studies were undertaken to specifically study the elderly population, but intrathecal (IT) delivery of opioids can be very useful in reducing cancer pain, from which older adults suffer more than the general population [70]. Krames recommends using IT analgesic therapy for patients with terminal, painful malignancies, whereas in those patients with less than 3 months to live, using a tunneled epidural catheter [71]. In his review, Erdine et al. concluded that intrathecal

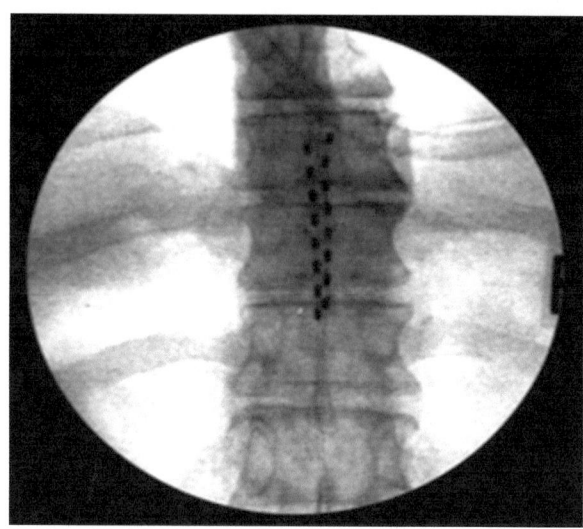

Fig. 11 Fluoroscopic image of percutaneous lead placement

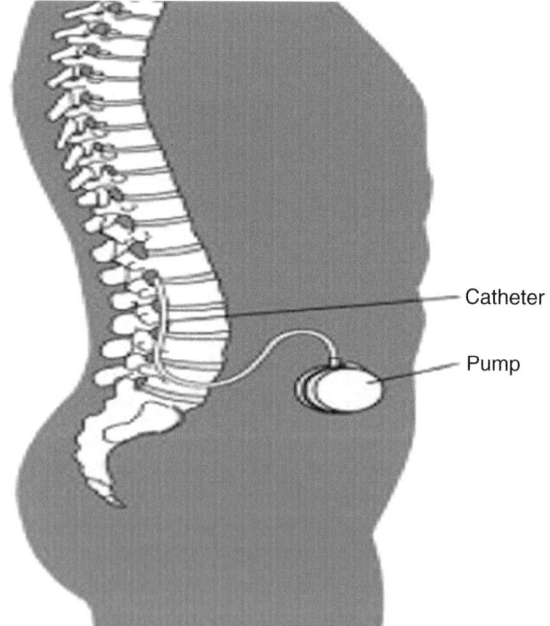

Fig. 12 Intrathecal analgesia pump system

drug delivery was an effective treatment in carefully selected patients with chronic pain that cannot be controlled by a well-tailored drug regime and/or spinal cord stimulation.

The SynchroMed® Infusion System from Medtronic is currently the only programmable, implantable pump on the market (Fig. 13). It became commercially available for the administration of intraspinal morphine for chronic pain in 1991.

Fig. 13 Medtronic SynchroMed II intrathecal pump. (Courtesy of Medtronic)

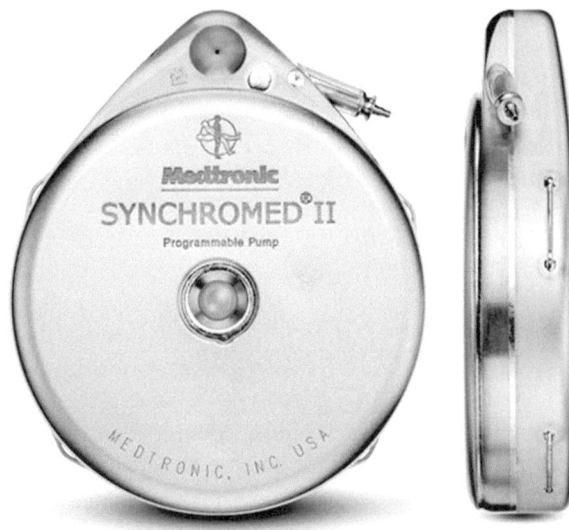

Table 3 Characteristics of patients with cancer who would benefit most from intrathecal analgesia

Patients with chronic intractable cancer pain
Patients suffering from advanced or recurrent cancers that typically metastasize to the bone, including breast, lung, colorectal, prostate, and head and neck cancer
Patients experiencing inadequate pain relief on ≥200 mg oral opioids per day or intolerable side effects on lower doses
Patients with a VAS ≥ 5
Patients receiving "round-the-clock" rather than p.r.n. dosing

VAS visual analogue score

The other intrathecal pump available is a Codman® pump that functions via a constant flow infusion technique. Results of the Cancer Pain Trial helped identify the type of patient with cancer who would benefit most from implantation of the SynchroMed® Infusion System [72]. Patients with the following characteristics would make ideal candidates: any patient with chronic intractable cancer pain; suffering from advanced or recurrent cancers that typically metastasize to the bone, including breast, lung, colorectal, prostate, and head and neck cancer; experiencing inadequate pain relief on ≥200 mg oral opioids per day or intolerable side effects on lower doses; with a VAS ≥ 5; and, at the time of their evaluation, receiving "round-the-clock" rather than p.r.n. dosing (Table 3). There are several absolute contraindications to implanting an infusion pump in the cancer pain population: tumor involvement that directly or indirectly encroaches on the intrathecal space that may inhibit the CSF flow necessary for effective analgesia with spinal administration; aplastic anemia characterized by pancytopenia, making the patient prone to infection and bleeding; and systemic or occult (obscure) infection which can lead to

Table 4 Contraindications to intrathecal analgesia delivery system

Absolute contraindications
Patient refusal
Tumor involvement directly or indirectly encroaching on intrathecal space
Aplastic anemia characterized by pancytopenia
Systemic or occult (obscure) infection
Relative contraindications
Emaciated patients who may not be able to support the weight of an implanted pump
Immune dysfunction
Thrombocytopenia
Malnutrition inhibiting proper healing
Decubiti as a source of infection

meningitis if it reaches the spinal column. Relative contraindications include emaciated patients who may not be able to support the weight of an implanted pump, immune dysfunction, thrombocytopenia, malnutrition inhibiting proper healing, and decubiti as a source of infection (Table 4) [73].

The evidence to support intrathecal systems for chronic nonmalignant pain is less robust than that for cancer pain and is controversial due to concerns of opioid-induced hyperalgesia, tolerance, and the potential for abuse [74]. In a systematic review of IT therapy for chronic noncancer pain, Patel et al. reported 15 observational studies that provide level II-3 or level III (based on the US Preventative Services Task Force criteria) evidence supporting the use of IT drug infusions for the treatment of chronic noncancer pain [75]. The British Pain Society published best practice recommendations on intrathecal systems and noted there was no RCT evidence but did observe supportive prospective open studies for chronic nonmalignant pain [76].

Complications of IT therapy include cerebrospinal fluid leak (with possible subsequent seroma formation), wound infection, hematoma, and granuloma formation at the catheter tip [77]. Potential drug-related side effects with long-term use of IT analgesics include nausea, constipation, pruritus, urinary retention, confusion, hypogonadism, and psychological disturbances [78]. In the older population, maintenance of an implantable drug delivery system can pose challenges due to transportation limitations to the clinic for IT pump medication refills. Alternatively, these refills now can be performed at home by specific home infusion providers (Christo et al. [6]).

Based on the current literature, IT analgesia should be considered primarily for those patients with cancer pain, with the possibility of careful selection regarding chronic nonmalignant pain.

Intra-articular Peripheral Joint Injections

Osteoarthritis (OA) is the most prevalent form of arthritis with a predicted 2020 prevalence as high as 18.2% of the US population [79]. Its prevalence increases with age, reaching approximately 68% of individuals aged 65 years or older. As a result of aging, it may occur in any joint, but the knee is most commonly affected and is a common cause of pain in the elderly. Knee pain decreases functional ability, thus strongly predicting future disability and dependency [80]. Common physical exam findings include pain on palpation, bony enlargement, crepitus on motion, and limited joint movement.

Intra-articular (IA) corticosteroid injections have been used for the treatment of OA for over 55 years [81]. A Cochrane review examined 26 RCTs comparing IA corticosteroids against placebo, IA hyaluronic acid (HA), and joint lavage [82]. The majority of patients in these trials were over the age of 50. The authors concluded that steroids were more effective than placebo in reducing pain in week 1 (NNT = 3–4). The effect continued for 3 weeks, but evidence afterward was poor. Intra-articular HA for pain relief in patients with knee pain from OA has increased in the last several decades. In another Cochrane review, Bellamy et al. concluded that viscosupplementation was efficacious in providing pain relief with beneficial effects on pain, function, and patient global assessment [83]. This treatment modality does not typically exert its benefits in pain reduction until after week 4 [84]. In general, the onset of effect is similar, but HA has more prolonged effects than IA corticosteroids [85].

Conclusion

Treating pain in the older patient can be a difficult task given the multiple comorbidities and age-specific factors that a patient in this age group may have. While pharmacotherapy is often utilized in managing pain, using interventions as part of a multimodal regimen that also includes medications, physical therapy, and cognitive-behavioral therapy provides an opportunity to reduce medication dosage and potential side effects. Several studies show promising results in the interventional treatment of pain in the elderly. However, there needs to be more robust prospective randomized controlled trials to better understand the impact these interventions have on the care of these patients.

References

1. Ozyalcin NS. Minimal invasive treatment modalities for geriatric pain management. Agri. 2004;16:26–36.
2. Freedman GM. Chronic pain. Clinical management of common causes of geriatric pain. Geriatrics. 2002;57:36–41.
3. Frymoyer JW, Cats-Baril WL. An overview of the incidence and costs of low back pain. Orthop Clin N Am. 1991;22:263–71.
4. Shamie AN. Lumbar spinal stenosis: the growing epidemic. AAOS Now. 2011;5(5):9–11.
5. Friedly J, Chan L, Deyo R. Increases in lumbosacral injections in the medicare population: 1994 to 2001. Spine (Phila Pa 1976). 2007;32(16):1754–60.
6. Christo PJ, Li S, Gibson SJ, Fine P, Hameed H. Effective treatments for pain in the older patient. Curr Pain Headache Rep. 2011;15(1):22–34.
7. Snyder DL, Doggartt D, Turkelson C. Treatment of degenerative lumbar spinal stenosis. Am Fam Physician. 2004;70:517–20.

8. Botwin K, Gruber R, Bouchlas CG, et al. Fluoroscopically guided lumbar transformational epidural steroid injections in degenerative lumbar stenosis. Am J Phys Med Rehabil. 2002;81:898–905.
9. Tadokoro K, Miyamoto H, Sumi M, Shimomura T. The prognosis of conservative treatments for lumbar stenosis: analysis of patients over 70 years of age. Spine. 2005;30:2458–63.
10. Koc Z, Ozcakir O, Sivrioglu K, Gurbet A, Kucukoglu S. Effectiveness of physical therapy and epidural steroid injections in lumbar spinal stenosis. Spine. 2009;34:985–9.
11. Shabat S, Folman Y, Leitner Y, Fredman B, Gepstein R. Failure of conservative treatment for lumbar stenosis in elderly patients. Arch Gerontol Geriatr. 2007;44:235–4.
12. Merskey H, Bogduk N. Classification of chronic pain: classifications of chronic pain descriptions of chronic pain syndromes and definitions of pain terms. 2nd ed. Seattle: IASP Press; 1994. p. 13–5.
13. Stafford MA, Peng P, Hill DA. Sciatica: a review of history, epidemiology, pathogenesis and the role of epidural steroid injection in management. BJA. 2010;99:461–73.
14. Weber H, Holme I, Amlie E. The natural course of acute sciatica with nerve root symptoms in a double-blind placebo-controlled trial evaluating the effect of piroxica. Spine. 1993;18:1433–8.
15. Lievre JA, Bloch-Michel H, Pean G. L'hydrocortisone en injection locale. Revue du Rhumatisme et des Maladies Osteo-articulares. 1953;20:310–1.
16. Watts RW, Silagy CA. A meta-analysis on the efficacy of epidural corticosteroids in the treatment of sciatica. Anaesth Intensive Care. 1995;23:564–9.
17. McQuay H, Moore A. Ch 27: epidural corticosteroids for sciatica. In: An evidenced based resource for pain relief. New York: Oxford University Press; 1998. p. 216–8.
18. Riew KD, Yuming Y, Gilula L, et al. The effect of nerve root injections on the need for operative treatment of lumbar radicular pain. J Bone Joint Surg Am. 2000;82:1589–3.
19. Bicket MC, Gupta A, Brown CH 4th, Cohen SP. Epidural injections for spinal pain: a systematic review and meta-analysis evaluating the "control" injections in randomized controlled trials. Anesthesiology. 2013;119(4):907–31.
20. Helbig T, Lee CK. The lumbar facet syndrome. Spine (Phila Pa 1976). 1988;13(1):61–4.
21. Cohen SP, Huang JH, Brummett C. Facet joint pain—advances in patient selection and treatment. Nat Rev Rheumatol. 2013;9(2):101–16.
22. Abdulla A, Adams N, Bone M, Elliott AM, Gaffin J, Jones D, et al. Guidance on the management of pain in older people. Age Ageing. 2013;42(Suppl 1):i1–57.
23. Manchikanti L, Pamapti V, Rivera J, Fellow B, Beyer C, Damron K. Role of facet joints in chronic back pain in the elderly: a controlled prevalence study. Pain Pract. 2001;1:332–7.
24. Manchikanti L, Manchikanti KN, Cash KA, Singh V, Giordano J. Age-related prevalence of facet-joint involvement in chronic neck and low back pain. Pain Physician. 2008;11:67–75.
25. Cohen SP, Raja SN. Pathogenesis, diagnosis and treatment of lumbar zygopophyseal (facet) joint pain. Anesthesiology. 2007;106:591–614.
26. van Kleef M, Vanelderen P, Cohen SP, Lataster A, Van Zundert J, Mekhail N. 12. Pain originating from the lumbar facet joints. Pain Pract. 2010;10(5):459–69.
27. van Kleef M, Barendse GA, Kessels A, Voets HM, Weber WE, de Lange S. Randomized trial of radiofrequency lumbar facet denervation for chronic low back pain. Spine (Phila Pa 1976). 1999;24(18):1937–42.
28. Leclaire R, Fortin L, Lambert R, Bergeron YM, Rossignol M. Radiofrequency facet joint denervation in the treatment of low back pain: a placebo-controlled clinical trial to assess efficacy. Spine (Phila Pa 1976). 2001;26(13):1411–6.
29. van Eerd M, Patijn J, Lataster A, et al. Cervical facet pain. Pain Pract. 2010;10:113–23.
30. Ward A, Watson J, Wood P, et al. Glucocorticoid epidural for sciatica: metabolic and endocrine sequelae. Rheumatology (Oxford). 2002;41(1):68–71.
31. Walker J. The sacroiliac joint: a critical review. Phys Ther. 1992;72:903–16.
32. Bernard TN, Cassidy JD. The sacroiliac syndrome. In: Frymoyer JW, editor. Pathophysiology, diagnosis and management. New York: Raven; 1991. p. 2107–30.
33. Bowen V, Cassidy JD. Macroscopic and microscopic anatomy of the sacroiliac joint from embryonic life until the eighth decade. Spine (Phila Pa 1976). 1981;6(6):620–8.

34. Vanelderen P, Szadek K, Cohen SP, De Witte J, Lataster A, Patijn J, et al. 13. Sacroiliac joint pain. Pain Pract. 2010;10(5):470–8.
35. Slipman CW, Jackson HB, Lipetz JS, et al. Sacroiliac joint pain referral zones. Arch Phys Med Rehabil. 2000;81(3):334–8.
36. Cohen SP. Sacroiliac joint pain: a comprehensive review of anatomy, diagnosis, and treatment. Anesth Analg. 2005;101:1440–53.
37. Cohen SP, Chen Y, Neufeld NJ. Sacroiliac joint pain: a comprehensive review of epidemiology, diagnosis and treatment. Expert Rev Neurother. 2013;13(1):99–116.
38. Kim WM, Lee HG, Jeong CW, Kim CM, Yoon MH. A randomized controlled trial of inta-articular prolotherapy versus steroid injection for sacroiliac joint pain. J Altern Complement Med. 2010;16(12):1285–90.
39. Luukkainen R, Nissila M, Asikainen E, et al. Periarticular corticosteroid treatment of the sacroiliac joint in patients with seronegative spondylarthropathy. Clin Exp Rheumatol. 1999;17(1):88–90.
40. Luukkainen RK, Wennerstrand PV, Kautiainen HH, Sanila MT, Asikainen EL. Efficacy of perirticular corticosteroi treatment of the sacroiliac joint in non-spondylarthropathic patients with chronic low back pain in the region of the sacroiliac joint. Clin Exp Rheumatol. 2002;20(1):52–4.
41. Rupert MP, Lee M, Manchikanti L, et al. Evaluation of sacroiliac joint interventions: a systematic appraisal of the literature. Pain Physician. 2009;12:399–418.
42. Johnell O, Kanis JA. An estimate of the worldwide prevalence and disability associated with osteoporotic fractures. Osteoporos Int. 2006;17(12):1726–33.
43. Bajaj S, Saag KG. Osteoporosis: evaluation and treatment. Curr Womens Health Rep. 2003;3(5):418–24.
44. Coper C, Atkinson EJ, O'Fallon WM, et al. Incidence of clinically diagnosed vertebral fractures: a population based study in Rochester, Minnesota, 1985–1989. J Bone Miner Res. 1993;7:221–7.
45. Jensen ME, McGraw JK, Cardella JF, Hirsch JA. Position statement on percutaneous vertebral augmentation: a consensus statement developed by the American Society of Interventional and Therapeutic Neuroradiology, Society of Interventional Radiology, American Association of Neurological Surgeons/Congress of Neurological Surgeons, and American Society of Spine Radiology. J NeuroInterv Surg. 2009;1:181–5.
46. Galibert P, Deramond H, Rosat P, et al. Preliminary note on the treatment of vertebral angioma by percutaneous acrylic vertebroplasty. Neurochirurgie. 1987;33(2):166–8.
47. Yu SW, Yang SC, Kao YH, Yen CY, Tu YK, Chen LH. Clinical evaluation of vertebroplasty for multiple-level osteoporotic spinal compression fracture in the elderly. Arch Orthop Trauma Surg. 2008;128:97–101.
48. Peh WCG, Gilula LA, Peck DD. Percutaneous vertebroplasty for severe osteoporotic vertebral body compression fractures. Radiology. 2002;223:121–6.
49. Mehbod A, Aunoble S, Le Huec JC. Vertebroplasty for osteoporotic spine fracture: prevention and treatment. Eur Spine J. 2003;12(Suppl 2):S155–62.
50. Lee BJ, Lee SR, Yoo TY. Paraplegia as a complication of percutaneous vertebroplasty with polymethylmethacrylate: a case report. Spine (Phila Pa 1976). 2002;27(19):E419–22.
51. Krueger A, Bliemel C, Zettl R, et al. Management of pulmonary cement embolism after percutaneous vertebroplasty and kyphoplasty: a systematic review of the literature. Eur Spine J. 2009;18(9):1257–65.
52. Do HM, Kim BS, Marcellus ML, Curtis L, Marks MP. Prospective analysis of clinical outcomes after percutaneous vertebroplasty for painful osteoporotic vertebral body fractures. AJNR Am J Neuroradiol. 2005;26:1623–8.
53. Voormolen MHJ, Mali WPTM, Lohle PNM, et al. Percutaneous vertebroplasty compared with optimal pain medication treatment: short-term clinical outcome of patients with subacute or chronic painful osteoporotic vertebral compression fractures. The vertos study. AJNR Am J Neuroradiol. 2007;28:555–60.

54. Layton KF, Thielen KR, Koch CA, et al. Vertebroplasty, first 1000 levels of a single center: evaluation of the outcomes and complications. AJNR Am J Neuroradiol. 2007;28:683–9.
55. Liliang PC, Su TM, Liang CL, Chen HJ, Tsai YD, Lu K. Percutaneous vertebroplasty improves pain and physical functioning in elderly osteoporotic vertebral compression fracture patients. Gerontology. 2005;51:34–9.
56. Klazen CA, Lohle PN, de Vries J, et al. Vertebroplasty versus conservative treatment in acute osteoporotic vertebral compression fractures (Vertos II): an open-label randomised trial. Lancet. 2010;376(9746):1085–92.
57. Wardlaw D, Cummings SR, Van Meirhaeghe J, et al. Efficacy and safety of balloon kyphoplasty compared with nonsurgical care for vertebral compression fracture (free): a randomised controlled trial. Lancet. 2009;373:1016–24.
58. Boonen S, Van Meirhaeghe J, Bastian L, Cummings SR, et al. Balloon kyphoplasty for the treatment of acute vertebral compression fractures: 2-year results from a randomized trial. J Bone Miner Res. 2011;26(7):1627–37.
59. Buchbinder R, Osborne RH, Ebeling PR, et al. Randomized trial of vertebroplasty for painful osteoporotic vertebral fractures. N Engl J Med. 2009;361:557–68.
60. Kallmes DF, Comstock BA, Heagerty PJ, et al. A randomized trial of vertebroplasty for osteoporotic spinal fractures. N Engl J Med. 2009;361:569–79.
61. Anderson PA, Froyshteter AB, Tontz WL Jr. Meta-analysis of vertebral augmentation compared with conservative treatment for osteoporotic spinal fractures. J Bone Miner Res. 2013;28(2):372–82.
62. Han S, Wan S, Ning L, et al. Percutaneous vertebroplasty versus balloon kyphoplasty for treatment of osteoporotic vertebral compression fracture: a meta-analysis of randomised and non-randomised controlled trials. Int Orthop. 2011;35:1349–58.
63. Shealy CN, Mortimer JT, Reswick JB. Electrical inhibition of pain by stimulation of the dorsal columns: preliminary clinical report. Anaesth Analg. 1967;46:489–91.
64. Melzack R, Wall PD. Pain mechanisms: a new theory. Science. 1965;150(699):971–9.
65. Deer T, Masone R. Selection of spinal cord stimulation candidates for the treatment of chronic pain. Pain Med. 2008;9(S1):S82–92.
66. Mekhail N, Aeshbach A, Stanton-Hicks M. Cost benefit analysis of neurostimulation for chronic pain. Clin J Pain. 2004;20(6):462–8.
67. North RB, Kidd DH, Farrokhi F, et al. Spinal cord stimulation versus repeated lumbosacral spine surgery for chronic pain: a randomized, controlled trial. Neurosurgery. 2005;56(1):98–106.
68. Kumar K, Taylor RS, Jacques L, et al. Spinal cord stimulation versus conventional medical management for neuropathic pain: a multicentre randomised controlled trial in patients with failed back surgery syndrome. Pain. 2007;132(1–2):179–88.
69. Pert CB, Snyder SH. Opiate receptor: demonstration in nervous tissue. Science. 1973;179(77):1011–4.
70. Hall S, Gallagher RM, Gracely E, et al. The terminal cancer patient: effects of age, gender, and primary tumor site on opioid dose. Pain Med. 2003;4(2):125–34.
71. Krames ES. Intrathecal infusional therapies for intractable pain: patient management guidelines. J Pain Symptom Manag. 1993;8(1):36–46.
72. Smith TJ, Staats PS, Deer T, Stearns LJ, Rauck RL, Boortz-Marx RL, Buchser E, Catala E, Bryce DA, Coyne PJ, et al. Randomized clinical trial of an implantable drug delivery system compared with comprehensive medical management for refractory cancer pain: impact on pain, drug-related toxicity, and survival. J Clin Oncol. 2002;20(19):4040–9.
73. Krames E. Clinical realities and economic considerations: patient selection in intrathecal therapy. J Pain Symptom Manag. 1997;14(3S):S3–S13.
74. Kalso E, Edwards JE, Moore RA, et al. Opioids in chronic noncancer pain: systematic review of efficacy and safety. Pain. 2004;112(3):372–80.
75. Patel VB, Manchikanti L, Singh V, et al. Systematic review of intrathecal infusion systems for long-term management of chronic non-cancer pain. Pain Physician. 2009;12(2):345–60.
76. The British Pain Society. Intrathecal drug delivery for the Management of Pain and Spasticity in adults; Recommendations for best practice. Prepared on behalf of the British Pain Society

in consultation with the Association for Palliative Medicine and the Society of British Neurological Surgeons. London: The British Pain Society, 2008.
77. Belverud S, Mogilner A, Schulder M. Intrathecal pumps. Neurotherapeutics. 2008;5(1):114–22.
78. Cohen SP, Dragovich A. Intrathecal analgesia. Anesthesiol Clin. 2007;25(4):863–82. viii
79. Lawrence RC, Helmick CG, Arnett FC, Deyo RA, Felson DT, Giannini EH, et al. Estimates of the prevalence of arthritis and selected musculoskeletal disorders in the United States. Arthritis Rheum. 1998;41:778–99.
80. Jinks C, Jordan K, Croft P. Osteoarthritis as a public health problem: the impact of developing knee pain on physical function in adults living in the community: (knest 3). Rheumatology. 2007;46:877–81.
81. Miller JH, White J, Norton TH. The value of intra-articular injections in osteoarthritis of the knee. J Bone Joint Surg Br. 1958;40:636–43.
82. Bellamy N, Campbell J, Robinson V, Gee TL, Bourne R, Wells G. Intraarticular corticosteroid for treatment of osteoarthritis of the knee. Cochrane Database Syst Rev. 2005;2:CD005328.
83. Bellamy N, Campbell J, Welch V, Gee TL, Bourne R, Wells GA. Viscosupplementation for the treatment of osteoarthritis of the knee. Cochrane Database Syst Rev. 2006;2:CD005321.
84. Modawal A, Ferrer M, Choi HK, Castle JA. Hyaluronic acid injections relieve knee pain. J Fam Pract. 2005;54:758–67.
85. Aggarwal A, Sempowski I. Hyaluronic acid injections for knee osteoarthritis. Systematic review of the literature. Can Fam Physician. 2004;50:249–56.

Assessing and Managing Addiction Risk in Older Adults with Pain

Steven D. Passik, Adam Rzetelny, and Kenneth Kirsh

Overview

Had this book appeared just a short decade or two ago, a chapter on the assessment and management of addiction risk in the older person with pain – if included at all – might have been included solely as a nod to completeness, and this chapter seen as somewhat *esoteric*. But it has been over this time period that the prescribing of opioids and other controlled substances has risen dramatically to treat chronic pain in our aging society. As this occurred, a public health crisis has arisen, the related problems of prescription drug abuse, diversion, overdose, and death. Eighty-five percent of addictions are manifest by the age of 35 [1]. An older person with a painful condition is unlikely to develop addiction de novo in the context of painful illness; however, increasing percentages of older Americans have a history of drug use in the remote or recent past. Furthermore, their medications may be sought after by younger drug abusers in their family who in turn are at risk for addiction, overdose, and death.

Thus, pain management in older people must begin with an appreciation of these risks (those related to their prior drug use history and those related to the potential for drug diversion) and proceed following upon a careful evaluation of risk for addiction and diversion with subsequent management strategies directed at identified risks. Though alcohol remains one of the most abused and problematic drugs in older adults, as in any age group, the focus of this chapter is the so-called hidden

S. D. Passik (✉)
Scientific Affairs, Education and Policy, Collegium Pharmaceuticals, Canton, MA, USA
e-mail: spassik@collegiumpharma.com

A. Rzetelny
Collegium Pharmaceuticals, Stoughton, MA, USA

K. Kirsh
Stoughton, MA, USA

Millennium Health of San Diego California, San Diego, CA, USA epidemic [2, 3] of illicit drugs and the misuse, abuse, and diversion of prescription medications among older adults.

Scope of the Problem and Trends

The belief that aging drug habits would diminish and vanish with age is no longer held as strongly as it once was. A 1962 study supporting this belief showed 50% of individuals addicted to narcotics were no longer active drug users by age 32 and over 99% were no longer users by age 67 [4]. However, as the "baby boom" cohort ages, the extent of alcohol and medication misuse is predicted to significantly increase because of the combined effect of the growing population of older adults and cohort-related differences in lifestyles and attitudes [5]. One study suggested that the number of drug users aged 50 years or older will approximately double from the year 2000 to the year 2020 because of an anticipated 52% increase in this segment of the population and the attendant shift in attitudes and historical experiences with substance use in this cohort [6].

The use of illicit drugs and nonmedical prescription opioids has increased significantly in the general population over the last decade [7] with the highest prevalence among younger adult men [8]. However, alarming trends are emerging among older adults. Currently, among adults aged 50 or older, nearly five million, or a little more than 5% of that age group, report using illicit drugs in the past year [9]. Marijuana is the most abused drug in the USA, but among adults aged 60 or older, the abuse of prescription drugs is equally common. A changing pattern of cannabis use among older adults suggests that as individuals age, the social incentive to smoke marijuana decreases, while the attempt to use it medicinally increases [2]. Emergency room visits related to pharmaceutical abuse more than doubled from 2004 to 2008 among adults aged 50 or older, and a fifth of these were among adults aged 70 or older [10]. Among these, prescription opioids were the most common, followed by benzodiazepines. Substance abuse treatment admissions among adults aged 50 and older have nearly doubled in recent years, from 6.6% of all admissions in 1992 to 12.7% in 2009 [11]. During this same time period, alcohol as the only substance of abuse being treated decreased from 87.6% to 58.0%, while the addition of other drugs to alcohol increased from 12.4% to 42.0%. Also around this time, treatment admissions involving heroin more than doubled, from 7.2% to 16.0%, and those reporting multiple drugs of abuse nearly tripled [12]. Although family and friends remain the most frequent sources of diverted prescription medications [1, 8], healthcare professionals are much more likely to represent the source of diversion among older adults in substance treatment settings (>60%) relative to younger adults (~30%) [1].

With the baby boomer population growing older and experiencing more pain, there is a paucity of information on older patients and the risk of comorbid pain and addiction. A survey in Denmark revealed that 22.5% of men and 27.8% of women aged 65 and older reported chronic pain [13]. Out of these men and women, 35% of them were not satisfied with the pain treatment that was offered.

This can lead to alternative methods for relieving pain such as taking nonprescribed medications. In one study of 100 patients with chronic pain (average age near 50), 23 tested positive for illicit drugs, and 12 tested positive for opioids even though they had no prescription and denied taking opioids [14]. In another study of primary care patients in a Veterans Affairs facility who were receiving opioids for the treatment of chronic pain (average age 59), 78% reported at least one indicator of medication misuse during the prior year, with significantly more of those who misused pain medications reporting comorbid substance use disorder [15]. This is consistent with a more recent examination of a subset of data from the Researched Abuse, Diversion and Addiction-Related Surveillance (RADARS) system that found that though severe chronic pain is common in adults entering treatment for prescription opioid abuse, it is exponentially more prevalent in adults older than 45 years (70%) relative to adults aged 18–24 (45%) [1]. Clearly, to the extent that chronic pain and substance abuse are comorbid or mutually exacerbating problems, older adults would appear to represent a particularly vulnerable population.

The emerging pattern, consistent with the aging of the "baby boom" generation and their greater likelihood of exposure to various types of drugs, is that illicit and prescription drug misuse and abuse, along with the need for treatment, are expected to double by 2020 (relative to 1990s prevalence estimates) among older adults [6, 16] with the greatest changes reflecting the increasing rates of emergency room visits and treatment admissions related to prescription opioids, benzodiazepines, heroin, and cocaine. Knowledge of these trends should assist providers in identifying and managing problems in a more age-appropriate manner.

Patterns

Roe and colleagues [17] described two general patterns of use by the elderly: "early-onset" and "late-onset" users. Early-onset users are more prevalent and have a long history of substance abuse and continue to abuse illicit drugs even as they age. Late-onset users, representing less than 10% of this population [2], are those who develop the habit when they are older (possibly in the context of medical exposures).

Late-onset substance abuse among the elderly is a less explored pattern. A variety of potential causes have been cited for such new-onset substance abuse. Table 1 lists possible causes.

Table 1 Potential causes of new-onset substance abuse in the elderly [18]

High rates of painful conditions
Self-medication
Depression
Dementia
Cognitive impairment
Social isolation
Poor support systems

Table 2 Risk factors for drug abuse in the elderly [3, 20–22]

Female gender
Social isolation
History of substance abuse
History of mental illness
Medical exposure to prescription drugs with abuse potential
Young elder (age 50–60)
Unmarried male
Low-income status
Current methadone maintenance
Substance abuse among close contacts
Involvement in crime, especially drug crime

Risk Factors

Unfortunately there are virtually no screening or assessment instruments available for identifying or diagnosing drug abuse that have been specifically validated in older adults [19]. Several factors may lead to increase risk and are outlined in Table 2.

Clinical Presentation

Prescribers need to know how to apply the principles and practices of addiction medicine to the care of all persons being treated with controlled substances, whether the patient is elderly or not. No one is immune to the risk of addiction [23–26].

As a first step in discussing how addiction presents clinically in older adults, it is first important to clarify what addiction is and is not. Addiction is not represented by physiological dependence, which is an expected development that follows upon continuous exposure (though the time period varies from days to weeks depending upon the person) to certain classes of drugs over time [27–29]. Dependence is not limited to pain medications but also occurs in response to corticosteroids, antidepressants, and even some blood pressure medications. Dependence refers to the fact that if a person abruptly stops a medicine in one of these classes, they will suffer with symptoms of withdrawal characteristic of that class of drugs. In the pain management setting, if a patient runs out of their opioid analgesics before they can get a refill from their doctor, they might suffer some symptoms of withdrawal, which include a flu-like syndrome, nervousness, excessive yawning, and goose bumps. The only important implications of the development of dependence are that if the person were to want to discontinue their medications, they would have to do it gradually and that it is important to take them as directed so they last between visits. Thus, dependence is not a sign that the pain patient is becoming addicted.

Addiction likewise is not based upon physiologic tolerance, which also is a normal development that follows upon continuous exposure (though the time period varies from days to weeks from person to person) to certain classes of drugs over time [29–31]. Tolerance refers to the need to increase the drug to maintain the desired effect, such as pain relief. The development of tolerance is highly variable in people with pain, and requests for higher doses need to be evaluated carefully. But, the need for some adjustment in dose over time is not a sign that the patient is becoming addicted. Importantly, because tolerance develops not only to the pain-relieving aspects of the drugs but also to side effects like sedation and the slowing down of one's breathing, the dose of opioids can be continually raised for patients suffering with progressive and debilitating conditions over time. Thus, misconceptions of tolerance often lead people to suffer because they are afraid that they need to save their pain medicines for when they really need them; such a practice is unnecessary.

Addiction is marked by the so-called 4Cs: craving, compulsive use, out of control use, and continued use despite harm [32, 33]. This definition appropriately emphasizes that addiction is, fundamentally, a psychological, neurological, and behavioral syndrome. While patients with addiction engage in aberrant and self-defeating behaviors, we must remember that aberrant behaviors may be indicative of one of several problems, and a differential diagnosis should be explored if questionable behaviors occur during pain treatment. While exposure to drugs is necessary, it is not sufficient to cause addiction. Addiction is the end result of a complex interaction between certain types of drugs and genetic, psychological, and stress vulnerabilities in the person. Aberrant behaviors such as unilateral dose escalation and subsequent requests for early prescription renewal can, for example, arise due to several forces; among them are poorly treated pain, self-medication of anxiety or depression, diversion by family members, true loss of control and addiction, or chemical coping in the face of life stressors.

In the medical setting, addiction issues will be identified by the 4Cs described above and identified by a growing set of aberrant behaviors being noted over time. Of specific note, clinicians should watch for signs of social withdrawal and worsening medical conditions, which might be indicative of an exacerbation of substance abuse. We will now discuss methods to begin an assessment process to identify these potentially aberrant behaviors.

Assessment

Pain management efforts must go on in a context of risk stratification and ongoing management. As part of this approach, prescribers can utilize brief screening tools when choosing candidates for such therapies and then engage in good charting techniques for ongoing assessment and management. This can be helpful for identifying patients that they can treat alone, those whom they can treat with help, and those whom they must refer to other specialists.

The assessment of substance use disorders (SUD) in older adults can be difficult due to a lack of instruments designed or validated for this population. Assessment tools utilized in younger populations likely have some utility but may lack sensitivity. For example, many screeners and assessment tools include items tapping legal consequences of substance abuse that are less common in older adults while at the same time lacking items related to accruing medical issues and loss of social networks more relevant for older populations. Most validated instruments for substance abuse in older adults are focused on alcohol, and some of these may be useful, though to a limited degree, for assessing other substances of abuse. Still, research related to Brief Intervention and Treatment for Elders (BRITE) shows that assessment options for the aged may be on the rise and provide unique utility.

An objective assessment tool widely utilized in settings where controlled substances are prescribed, and an important component of universal precautions, is urine or oral fluid testing (henceforth referred to as urine drug testing (UDT)). UDT is initially an assessment tool but becomes part of ongoing monitoring during the management phase. Nearly universally, various associations, organizations, and government agencies, such as the American Pain Society, American Society of Addiction Medicine, Federation of State Medical Boards, Substance Abuse and Mental Health Services Administration, and National Institutes of Health, to name a few, recommend the use of UDT for assessing and managing the risks associated with controlled substance misuse, abuse, and diversion. A number of studies suggest the prevalence of unexpected UDTs (toxicology results that show the presence of an illicit substance, the presence of a medication not prescribed, or an absence of a prescribed medication) in pain practices ranges from 30% to 45% [34, 35]. Data from these same studies indicate that clinicians are imperfect at detecting these problems in their patients, even when they are experienced at detecting aberrant behaviors, and generally underestimate the prevalence of unexpected UDTs.

In older people with pain, urine drug test results may indicate a variety of issues not limited to drug abuse by the patient themselves. In our clinical experience, UDT sometimes gave the first indication of problems in the elder abuse spectrum. We have seen examples of older patients who tested negative for a prescribed medication, and upon review with the patient, it was ultimately found that family members were stealing the medication and/or specifically threatening the patient with violence if they did not continue to complain of pain to their physician to obtain medications for their continued diversion. Given the widely held myth that older adults do not abuse their medications or illicit substances, and the data to the contrary, it is important to emphasize the need for monitoring in older populations.

In thinking about utilizing risk assessments, some thought needs to be given toward how they are implemented and introduced to patients. On one hand, many patients at low risk for abuse are fearful of becoming addicted to opioids and asking questions about addiction could heighten their anxiety [36]. For these patients, using screening tools can be turned into a way of reassuring them that they indeed do not have a history suggestive of risk. On the other hand, many patients will be fearful that acknowledging substance use or abuse might lead to a lack of treatment in general and lack of access to opioids in particular. While the incentive to lie may be quite high, the clinician needs to assure patients that no one set pattern of answers automatically leads to a denial and to introduce the screening process as a way of helping to plan for safe opioid treatment.

Given time constraints, time-sensitive measures are clearly needed to help in establishing risk stratification for the elderly patient with pain issues. The acknowledgment of this need has led to a substantial increase in addiction-related screening tools [37]. Many screening tools contain items on personal and family history of addiction as well as other history-related risk factors, such as preadolescent sexual abuse, age, and psychological disease. Some of the tools are particular to pain management, whereas others simply assess risk factors for addiction in general. While there is merit to having some form or risk assessment, it must be noted that it is unclear exactly which assessment tools ultimately provide the best results [38]. Whatever tool the clinician chooses, it is advised that he or she presents the screening process to the patient with the assurance that there are no answers that will negatively influence effective pain management.

There has been a growing interest in the development of tools that can be useful for screening patients up front to determine relative risk for patients having problems with prescription drug abuse or misuse, although as mentioned earlier little has been done to validate these on older adults to date. Regarding brief screening instruments, a number have arisen, including the Screening Tool for Addiction Risk (STAR), Drug Abuse Screening Test (DAST), Screener and Opioid Assessment for Patients with Pain (SOAPP), and Opioid Risk Tool (ORT), among others [39–42]. The choice in tools for more thorough ongoing assessment, however, has been somewhat more limited traditionally.

For longer-term assessment and updates, it is important to consider four main domains in assessing pain outcomes with an eye toward identifying addiction or misuse behaviors: (1) pain relief, (2) functional outcomes, (3) side effects, and (4) drug-related behaviors. These domains have been labeled the "4 A's" (analgesia, activities of daily living, adverse effects, and aberrant drug-related behaviors) for teaching purposes [43]. The Pain Assessment and Documentation Tool (PADT) was designed as a simple charting device based upon the 4 A's concept. It was designed to focus on key outcomes and provide a consistent way to document progress in pain management therapy over time while being intuitive, pragmatic, and adaptable to clinical situations [44, 45].

Interviews

Along with screening efforts, the interview process should not be overlooked. Although demographics should be examined from the history and physical intake, specific risk factors such as age at first use might be more indicative of problems with substances such as tobacco as opposed to opioids [46–49]. In an effort to not offend, threaten, or anger patients, clinicians many times avoid asking patients about drug abuse. There is also often the expectation that patients will not answer truthfully. However, obtaining a detailed history of duration, frequency, and desired effect of drug use is vital. Adopting a nonjudgmental position and communicating in an empathetic and truthful manner are the best strategy when taking patients' substance abuse histories [50, 51].

In anticipating defensiveness on the part of the patient, it can be helpful for clinicians to mention that patients often misrepresent their drug use for logical reasons, such as stigmatization, mistrust of the interviewer, or concerns regarding fears of undertreatment. It is also wise for clinicians to explain that in an effort to keep the patient as comfortable as possible, by preventing withdrawal states and prescribing sufficient medication for pain and symptom control, an accurate account of drug use is necessary [50, 51].

The use of a careful, graduated-style interview can be beneficial in slowly introducing the assessment of drug abuse. This approach begins with broad and general inquiries regarding the role of drugs in the patient's life, such as caffeine and nicotine, and gradually proceeds to more specific questions regarding illicit drugs. This interview style can also assist in discerning any coexisting psychiatric disorders, which can significantly contribute to aberrant drug-taking behavior. Once identified, treatment of comorbid psychiatric disorders can greatly enhance management strategies and decrease the risk of relapse [50, 51].

Management/Treatment/Prevention

Given the growth of the elderly segment of the population and the concomitant rise of substance abuse (SA) among them [6], including substance use disorders (SUD), we expect the need for treatment to steadily increase. Though the treatment of alcohol abuse represents the greatest proportion of the substance abuse treatment literature and is reviewed elsewhere (for a list of related publications, see the National Institute on Alcohol Abuse and Alcoholism (NIAAA) http://www.niaaa.nih.gov/), the focus in this section and throughout this chapter is on the emerging problem of illicit and prescription drug abuse or the so-called "hidden" or "silent" epidemic [2, 3]. As abuse of illicit and prescription drugs among older adults is on the rise, enhanced efforts aimed at identifying and treating non-alcohol substance abuse are needed [3]. Because of their disproportionate and expanding presence in varied medical settings, pain specialty settings being chief among them, and the increasing likelihood that comorbid substance abuse problems will initially present in these settings, combined with potentially limited access to specialty treatment, it is incumbent upon primary healthcare and other medical professionals to embrace their increasing role as the "front line" in addressing this problem. This involves greater awareness of prevalence, risks, and patterns that can lead to proactive identification and being ready with age-appropriate management and treatment responses, including a risk-stratified approach to identifying which individuals can be managed in the primary healthcare setting, co-managed, or referred to specialty treatment.

There is a dearth of information on the challenges of treatment for elderly drug abusers. Most treatments are geared toward young adults who comprise the majority of drug abusers. There has been data that show certain factors significant for treatment in young adults have been able to apply to the elderly as well. Pope [52] noted that family participation remains significant even into older adulthood.

There are several support groups for elderly adults that are specific to alcoholism (Seniors in Sobriety), but few are specific for illicit drugs. Interestingly, the Primary

Care Research in Substance Abuse and Mental Health for the Elderly study demonstrated no difference in efficacy in the treatment of elderly alcoholics between those receiving brief intervention sessions at primary care clinics and those receiving treatment at mental health or substance abuse clinics [53].

As noted above, the awareness that elderly patients have increased pharmacokinetic sensitivity and concomitantly greater susceptibility to adverse effects of many substances should also be included in substance abuse treatment. In part due to known genetic variability of drug-metabolizing enzymes [54], the metabolism of drugs can differ from patient to patient and can become problematic when installing a treatment plan for drug abusers. Awareness of potential drug-drug interactions associated with specific hepatic metabolism is especially critical in this population. Comorbid diseases can also affect the metabolism of drugs, such as diabetes or kidney disease, both being more prevalent among older adults [55]. It is recommended that when beginning substance abuse treatment with the elderly one start with lower doses and titrate slowly. Analogously, this may be true as well for behavioral interventions (i.e., cognitive-behavioral or brief interventions) in which lower intensity regiments may be more effective among older populations [21].

Risk-Stratified Management and Treatment

As noted above, risk management typically involves "universal precautions" [56, 57]. Such precautions will likely be applied similarly in elderly and non-elderly populations but may be enhanced if tailored to the specific needs of older adults. Risk stratification is part of every assessment and reassessment phase of treatment. Patients with a known history of substance abuse have elevated risk, but for older adults, understanding the entire clinical picture is critical. For example, late-onset substance abusers may respond adequately to simple education and monitoring strategies, whereas early-onset abusers will likely require a more comprehensive approach [17]. Additionally, there may be greater fear and reluctance to admit drug problems or accept help among older adults [1]. In all cases, once an older patient has been appropriately assessed and his or her degree of risk ascertained, management begins with frank and nonjudgmental communication with the patient about the potential risks and benefits of various treatments, including the risks of misuse, abuse, and diversion associated with controlled substances. It is worth bearing in mind that healthcare practitioners (HCPs) are much more likely than dealers to be the source of diversion among older adults relative to younger adults [1], and education should include safe storage and disposal of controlled substances.

Communication and education about the risks and benefits comprise part of informed consent and should be codified as part of an individualized treatment agreement [58, 59]. The cognitive status of the older patient must be taken into account when estimating his or her ability to understand and remember such education or for self-report of medication adherence, changes in disease state, or functioning. In some cases, inclusion of family members involved in the patient's treatment should be considered. The treatment agreement is also an opportunity to let older patients know what to expect and what is expected of them. For example, such agreements will often announce that (a) a baseline UDT toxicology and other forms of monitoring will be performed and repeated periodically (at a rate deemed appropriate by the HCP and based on the patient's level of risk), (b) dose escalations or other changes cannot be made without consultation with the healthcare provider, and (c) coordination with other healthcare providers will occur and that all prescriptions must be accurately reported to the HCP and filled at a single pharmacy. They should also be informed of the risks of concomitant illicit drug use if appropriate. For patients with a known history of illicit substance abuse but who are currently abstinent, that abstinence can be a condition of treatment. The consequences of deviating from the treatment agreement can also be incorporated. Deviations from the treatment agreement, as well as other aberrant behaviors and changes in risk assessments, may warrant escalation of monitoring, increasing the frequency of prescriptions while reducing their quantities, switching to medications or formulations with lowered abuse liability, and potentially co-managing with addiction specialists. In such cases, having a pre-established relationship with a professional who specializes in treating substance use disorders can be enormously helpful and provides the ability to offer a legitimate referral should the need arise.

As noted earlier, pain and primary healthcare providers will frequently represent the "front line" in identifying and intervening in substance abuse among this population. The Consensus Panel of the Treatment Improvement Protocol (TIP) has recommended that, in addition to screening in medical settings, the least intensive treatment modalities be attempted initially, including motivational interviewing and other nonconfrontational and supportive interventions [60, 61]. Consistent with these recommendations, screening, brief intervention, and referral to treatment (SBIRT; Substance Abuse and Mental Health Services Administration {SAMHSA} TIP 26; SAMHSA TIP 34) is a well validated model that may provide particular utility for dealing with potential substance abuse problems in older adults. Because substance abuse among older adults has been referred to as the "silent epidemic" [3], SBIRT may be especially apt for this population because it is predicated on universal screening, allowing healthcare professionals to identify and respond appropriately to these health problems in individuals who may be reluctant to admit or may not be actively seeking treatment for substance abuse. The majority of evidence supports the use of SBIRT for alcohol and tobacco, but data is accumulating regarding efficacy for illicit and prescription drug abuse, including opioids, cocaine, heroin, and amphetamine [62–64]. The Substance Abuse and Mental Health Services Administration (SAMHSA) defines the basic components of SBIRT:

- It is brief (e.g., typically about 5–10 min for brief interventions, about 5–12 sessions for brief treatments).
- The screening is universal.
- One or more specific behaviors related to risky alcohol and drug use are targeted.
- The services occur in a public health non-substance abuse treatment setting.
- It is comprehensive (comprised of screening, brief intervention/treatment, and referral to treatment).

Screening involves risk stratification using brief validated tools described above in the assessment section. At a minimum, a tool such as the CAGE (a four question questionnaire for screening for alcohol abuse), adapted for potential illicit or prescription substance abuse, may be appropriate as it is particularly brief and entirely verbal, conducted during an interview or in the course of impromptu conversation. The goal of brief intervention (5–10 min) is to educate patients and increase their motivation to reduce risky behavior. The goal of brief treatment (which usually involves 5–12 sessions) is not only to change the immediate behavior or thoughts about a risky behavior but also to address long-standing problems and help steer patients toward higher levels of care, potentially involving appropriate referral. Motivational interviewing is the cornerstone of brief interventions and some treatments, and some of its components include a nonjudgmental and collaborative stance with the patient, active and reflective listening, and developing and building on a patient's strengths and goals rather than merely focusing on their weaknesses and problems [65]. Establishing strong referral linkages in advance is critical, and a relative lack of appropriate referral sources can be an obstacle in some areas. Nevertheless, the Screening, Brief Intervention and Referral to Treatment (SBIRT) is intended to be brief and simple enough that it can be implemented by various healthcare providers, such as physicians, nurse practitioners, nurses, physician assistants, and social workers, in a variety of busy healthcare settings, e.g., emergency rooms, primary care offices, pain clinics, and residential facilities. Moreover, SBIRT is billable in many instances when providers are properly trained and certified, a process that can require only a day in some cases.

Recent preliminary evidence suggests that an adaptation of SBIRT tailored for older adults (the Florida Brief Intervention and Treatment for Elders [BRITE] project) may enhance substance abuse outcomes in this population [66]. The BRITE project is based on the SAMHSA model of SBIRT [60, 67] and included the development of protocols, workbooks, and outcome data. Consistent with features of older populations dealing with potential substance abuse issues, the BRITE project differed from other SBIRT programs largely through outreach and delivery of services to older adults where they live and receive services. It also emphasizes screening of medication use, both over-the-counter (OTC) and prescription, as well as highly prevalent comorbid depression. Interventions are at times delivered at patients' homes or residential facilities, and an age-appropriate flexibility is incorporated that considers patients' potentially altered cognitive status and fatigability, at times requiring interventions of shorter durations. Some encouraging, though preliminary, outcome data include reductions at discharge in prescription medication misuse (32%), OTC misuse (95.8%), and illicit drug use (75.0%).

Prevention

It has been argued that third-party payers are increasingly more likely to cover medical conditions that may be associated with substance abuse rather than the substance abuse per se, potentially contributing to the trend for substance abuse among older adults to be identified and managed in non-substance treatment settings. Though this may create conditions that are more economical for hospitals and patients to address the secondary and comorbid conditions associated with substance abuse, this is not necessarily the most effective strategy for optimizing treatment for patients or for costs to society [1]. Thus, a case for an increasing need for prevention can be made. Fortunately, with its emphasis on early, proactive identification of mental health and substance abuse problems, SBIRT, and in particular BRITE with its community outreach components, provides the additional potential benefit of prevention. As noted above, substance abuse among older adults has been described as the "silent epidemic," reflecting, potentially, a greater reluctance to report SA, fewer opportunities secondary to economic obstacles and medically related mobility issues, reduced social networks, and potentially compromised cognitive status. Given that this problem is expected to increase rapidly in the coming years [6], prevention may represent a critical and cost-effective step toward mitigating this trend.

Consistent with these goals, and the outcomes of the BRITE project, Zanjani and colleagues [68] examined the effectiveness of the Mental Healthiness and Aging Initiative (MHAI) intervention, a rural community educational outreach program aimed at raising awareness of mental health and substance abuse problems among the elderly population. Much of the work involved in this project involved identifying, recruiting, and organizing existing community resources across diverse and widely distributed geographies in the State of Kentucky. By providing proactive, universal education, this model represents a relatively inexpensive and effective model of the prevention of substance abuse among older adults. Though their findings were mixed and need to be replicated in other older populations, the results were encouraging, with many instances of awareness of relevant problems being maintained at 3 and 6 months. More importantly, the MHAI and BRITE projects demonstrate the viability and potential efficacy of prevention efforts that utilize coordinated, age-appropriate community outreach.

Summary and Conclusion

Pain treatment in the older patient must begin with an appreciation for the risks of drug abuse and diversion that have grown in recent years. While there is a lack of data pertaining to the components of a risk management paradigm in general and specifically to how it applies to the older patient with pain, a clinician can and should apply techniques and tools that have shown promise in the management of the younger person with pain. Some clinicians might view some of the foregoing as "overkill." In the end though, our duty to treat pain safely and effectively for the patient and to do so in a way that also protects the community against diversion mandates that elements of this approach be adopted. In the end, when done well, this approach may lead to satisfying outcomes even in some highly challenging clinical situations.

Addiction, addiction risk, and diversion are issues that need to be addressed if a prescriber determines that a potentially addicting medication is going to be used for pain management. Everyone has potential risk. If a clinician is going to prescribe medications with potential addiction risk, there needs to be:

- A clear goal for the use of the addicting medication
- Evaluation of the risk for addiction
- Discussion of the risk of addiction with the patient
- An opioid agreement with the patient about how the medication will be used and stopped
- Ongoing evaluation of addiction development
- Ongoing evaluation of effect of pain medication on pain and function
- Appropriate documentation of the use of the medication and its effect

References

1. Cicero TJ, Surratt HL, Kurtz S, Ellis MS, Inciardi JA. Patterns of prescription opioid abuse and co-morbidity in an aging treatment population. J Subst Abus Treat. 2012;42(1):87–94.
2. Taylor, M. H.; Grossberg, G. T. The growing problem of illicit substance abuse in the elderly: a review. Prim Care Companion CNS Disord 2012, 14(4).
3. Wu LT, Blazer DG. Illicit and nonmedical drug use among older adults: a review. J Aging Health. 2011;23:481–504.
4. Winick C. Maturing out of narcotic addiction. Bull Narc. 1962;14:1–7.
5. Patterson TL, Jeste DV. The potential impact of the baby-boom generation on substance abuse among elderly persons. Psychiatr Serv. 1999;50(9):1184–8.
6. Colliver JD, Compton WM, Gfroerer J, Condon T. Projecting drug use among aging baby boomers in 2020. Ann Epidemiol. 2006;16:257–65.
7. Manchikanti L, Singh A. Therapeutic opioids: a ten-year perspective on the complexities and complications of the escalating use, abuse, and nonmedical use of opioids. Pain Phys. 2008;11:S63–8.
8. SAMHSA. Results from the 2012 national survey on drug use and health: summary of national findings. Rockville: Substance Abuse and Mental Health Services Administration; 2013.
9. SAMHSA. National survey on drug use and health: illicit drug use among older adults. Rockville: Substance Abuse and Mental Health Services Administration (SAMHSA); 2011.
10. SAMHSA. Drug abuse warning network: emergency department visits involving illicit drug use by older adults: 2008. Rockville: Substance Abuse and Mental Health Services Administration; 2010.
11. SAMHSA. Treatment Episode Data Set (TEDS): older adult admissions reporting alcohol as a substance of abuse: 1992 and 2009, Substance Abuse and Mental Health Services Administration. 2011.
12. SAMHSA. Treatment Episode Data Set (TEDS). Changing substance abuse patterns among older admissions: 1992 and 2008. Rockville: Substance Abuse and Mental Health Services Administration; 2010.
13. Sjorgren P, Okholm O, Peuckmann V, Gronbaek M. Epidemiology of chronic pain in Denmark: an update. Eur J Pain. 2009;13:287–92.

14. Manchikanti L, Damron KS, McManus CD, Barnhill RC. Patterns of illicit drug use and opioid abuse in patients with chronic pain at initial evaluation: a prospective, observational study. Pain Phys. 2004;7:431–7.
15. Morasco B, Dobscha S. Prescription medication misuse in substance use disorder in VA primary care patients with chronic pain. Gen Hosp Psychiatry. 2008;30:93–9.
16. Gfroerer J, Penne M, Pemberton M, Folsom R. Substance abuse treatment need among older adults in 2020: the impact of the aging baby-boom cohort. Drug Alcohol Depend. 2003;69(2):127–35.
17. Roe B, Beynon C, Pickering L, Duffy P. Experience of drug use and ageing: health, quality of life, relationships and service implications. J Adv Nurs. 2010;66(9):1968–79.
18. Arndt S, Turvey CL, Flaum M. Older offenders, substance abuse, and treatment. Am J Geriatr Psychiatry. 2002;10(6):733–9.
19. Culberson JW, Ziska M. Prescription drug misuse/abuse in the elderly. Geriatrics. 2008;63(9):22–6.
20. Simoni-Wastila L, Yang HK. Psychoactive drug abuse in older adults. Am J Geriatr Pharmacother. 2006;4(4):380–94.
21. Briggs WP, Magnus VA, Lassiter P, Patterson A, Smith L. Substance use, misuse, and abuse among older adults: implications for clinical mental health counselors. J Ment Health Couns. 2011;33(2):112–27.
22. Rosen D, Hunsaker A, Albert SM, Cornelius JR, Reynolds CF. Characteristics and consequences of heroin use among older adults in the United States: a review of literature, treatment implications, and recommendations for further research. Addict Behav. 2011;36(4):279–85.
23. Grant BF, Dawson DA. Age at onset of alcohol use and its association with DSM-IV alcohol abuse and dependence: results from the National Longitudinal Alcohol Epidemiologic Survey. J Subst Abus. 1997;9:103–10.
24. Hingson RW, Heeren T, Winter MR. Age of alcohol-dependence onset: associations with severity of dependence and seeking treatment. Pediatrics. 2006;118:755–63.
25. Volkow ND. What do we know about drug addiction? Am J Psychiatr. 2005;162(8):1401–2.
26. Volkow ND, Li TK. Drugs and alcohol: treating and preventing abuse, addiction and their medical consequences. Pharmacol Ther. 2005;108(1):3–17.
27. Dole VP. Narcotic addiction, physical dependence and relapse. N Engl J Med. 1972;286:988–91.
28. Martin WR, Jasinski DR. Physiological parameters of morphine dependence in man tolerance, early abstinence, protracted abstinence. J Psychiatr Res. 1969;7:9–13.
29. Schneider J, Kirsh KL. Defining clinical issues around tolerance, hyperalgesia and addiction: a quantitative and qualitative outcome study of long-term opioid dosing in a chronic pain practice. J Opioid Manag. 2010;6(6):385–95.
30. Candiotti KA, Gitlin MC. Review of the effect of opioid-related side effects on the undertreatment of moderate to severe chronic non-cancer pain: tapentadol, a step toward a solution? Curr Med Res Opin. 2010;26(7):1677–84.
31. Noble M, Treadwell JR, Tregear SJ, Coates VH, Wiffen PJ, Akafomo C, Schoelles KM. Long-term opioid management for chronic noncancer pain. Cochrane Database Syst Rev. 2010;20(1):CD006605.
32. ASAM. ASAM public policy statement: The definition of addiction; American Society of Addiction Medicine. 2011.
33. Rinaldi RC, Steindler EM, Wilford BB, Goodwin D. Clarification and standardization of substance abuse terminology. J Amer Med Assoc. 1988;259(4):555–7.
34. Katz NP, Sherburne S, Beach M, Rose RJ, Vielguth J, Bradley J, Franciullo GJ. Behavioral monitoring and urine toxicology testing in patients receiving long-term opioid therapy. Anesth Analg. 2003;97:1097–102.
35. Michna E, Jamison RN, Pham LD, Ross EL, Janfaza D, Nedeljkovic SS, Narang S, Palombi D, Wasan AD. Urine toxicology screening among chronic pain patients on opioid therapy: frequency and predictability of abnormal findings. Clin J Pain. 2007;23:173–9.
36. Passik SD, Kirsh KL, McDonald MV, Ahn S, Russak SM, Martin L, Rosenfeld B, Breitbart WS, Portenoy RK. A pilot survey of aberrant drug-taking attitudes and behaviors in samples of cancer and AIDS patients. J Pain Symptom Manag. 2000;19:274–86.

37. Passik SD, Kirsh KL, Casper D. Addiction-related assessment tools and pain management: instruments for screening, treatment planning, and monitoring compliance. Pain Med. 2008;9(S2):145–66.
38. Chou R, Fanciullo GJ, Fine PG, Miaskowski C, Passik SD, Portenoy RK. Opioids for chronic noncancer pain: prediction and identification of aberrant drug-related behaviors: a review of the evidence for an American Pain Society and American Academy of Pain Medicine Clinical Practice Guideline. J Pain. 2009;10:131–46.
39. Butler SF, Budman SH, Fernandez K, Jamison RN. Validation of a screener and opioid assessment measure for patients with chronic pain. Pain. 2004;112(1–2):65–75.
40. Friedman R, Li V, Mehrotra D. Treating pain patients at risk: evaluation of a screening tool in opioid-treated pain patients with and without addiction. Pain Med. 2003;4(2):182–5.
41. Gavin DR, Ross HE, Skinner HA. Diagnostic validity of the drug abuse screening test in the assessment of DSM-III drug disorders. Br J Addict. 1989;84(3):301–7.
42. Webster LR, Webster RM. Predicting aberrant behaviors in opioid-treated patients: preliminary validation of the opioid risk tool. Pain Med. 2005;6(6):432–42.
43. Passik SD, Weinreb HJ. Managing chronic nonmalignant pain: overcoming obstacles to the use of opioids. Adv Ther. 2000;17:70–83.
44. Passik SD, Kirsh KL, Whitcomb LA, Portenoy RK, Katz N, Kleinman L, Dodd S, Schein J. A new tool to assess and document pain outcomes in chronic pain patients receiving opioid therapy. Clin Ther. 2004;26(4):552–61.
45. Passik SD, Kirsh KL, Whitcomb LA, Schein JR, Kaplan M, Dodd S, Kleinman L, Katz NP, Portenoy RK. Monitoring outcomes during long-term opioid therapy for non-cancer pain: results with the pain assessment and documentation tool. J Opioid Manag. 2005;1(5):257–66.
46. Benowitz NL. Pharmacology of nicotine: addiction and therapeutics. Annu Rev Pharmacol Toxicol. 1996;36:597–613.
47. Blum K, Braverman ER, Holder JM. Reward deficiency syndrome: A biogenetic model for the diagnosis and treatment of impulsive, addictive, and compulsive behaviors. J Psychoactive Drugs. 2000;32(Supplement:i–iv):1–112.
48. Breslau N, Johnson EO, Hiripi E, Kessler R. Nicotine dependence in the United States: prevalence, trends, and smoking persistence. Arch Gen Psychiatry. 2001;58(9):810–6.
49. Giovino GA, Henningfield JE, Tomar SL, Escobedo LG, Slade J. Epidemiology of tobacco use and dependence. Epidemiol Rev. 1995;17(1):48–65.
50. Passik SD, Portenoy RK. Substance abuse disorders. In: Psycho-oncology. New York: Oxford University Press; 1998. p. 576–86.
51. Savage SR, Kirsh KL, Passik SD. Challenges in using opioids to treat pain in persons with substance use disorders. Addict Sci Clin Pract. 2008;4(2):4–25.
52. Pope RC, Wallhagen M, Davis H. The social determinants of substance abuse in African American baby boomers: effects of family, media images, and environment. J Transcult Nurs. 2010;21(3):246–56.
53. Oslin DW, Grantham S, Coakley E, Maxwell J, Miles K, Ware J, Blow FC, Krahn DD, Bartels SJ, Zubritsky C, Olsen E, Kirchner JE, Levkoff S. Comparison of integrated care and enhanced specialty referral in managing at-risk alcohol use. Psychiatr Serv. 2006;57(7):954–8.
54. Gudin J. Opioid therapies and cytochrome P450 interactions. J Pain Symptom Manag. 2012;10(5):S4–S14.
55. Ondus KA, Hujer ME, Mann AE, Mion LC. Substance abuse and the hospitalized elderly. Orthop Nurs. 1999;18(4):27–36.
56. Gourlay DL, Heit HA. Universal precautions in pain medicine: a rational approach to the treatment of chronic pain. Pain Med. 2005;6:107.
57. Gourlay D, Heit H. Universal precautions: a matter of mutual trust and responsibility. Pain Med. 2006;7(2):210–2.
58. SAMHSA. Managing chronic pain in adults with or in recovery from substance use disorders. HHS Publication No. (SMA) 12–4671. Treatment Improvement Protocol (TIP) Series 54. Rockville: Substance Abuse and Mental Health Services Administration; 2011.

59. Peppin JF, Passik SD, Couto JE, Fine PG, Christo PJ, Argoff C, Aronoff GM, Bennett D, Cheatle MD, Slevin KA, Goldfarb NI. Recommendations for urine drug monitoring as a component of opioid therapy in the treatment of chronic pain. Pain Med. 2012;13:886–96.
60. Center for Substance Abuse Treatment. Substance abuse among older adults; Treatment Improvement Protocol (TIP) Series 26. Rockville, MD: Substance Abuse and Mental Health Services Administration, US Dept of Health and Human Services; DHHS publication no. SMA 98–3179. Rockville: Substance Abuse and Mental Health Services Administration; 1998.
61. Center for Substance Abuse Treatment. Substance abuse relapse prevention for older adults: a group treatment approach. Rockville: Substance Abuse and Mental Health Services Administration; 2005.
62. Cunningham R, Bernstein S, Walton M, Broderick K, Vaca F, Woolard R, Bernstein E, Blow F, D'Onofrio G. Alcohol, tobacco, and other drugs: future directions for screening and intervention in the emergency department. Acad Emerg Med. 2009;16:1078–88.
63. Madras BK, Compton WM, Avula D, Stegbauer T, Stein JB, Clark HW. Screening, brief interventions, referral to treatment (SBIRT) for illicit drug and alcohol use at multiple healthcare sites: comparison at intake and 6 months later. Drug Alcohol Depend. 2009;99(1–3):280–95.
64. WHO. The effectiveness of a brief intervention for illicit drugs linked to the alcohol, smoking, and substance involvement screening test (ASSIST) in 30 primary health care settings: a technical report of phase III findings of the WHO ASSIST Randomized control; World Health Organization. 2008.
65. Center for Substance Abuse Treatment. Enhancing Motivation for Change in Substance Abuse Treatment; Treatment Improvement Series (TIP) 35. Rockville: Substance Abuse and Mental Health Services Administration; 1999.
66. Schonfeld L, King-Kallimanis BL, Duchene DM, Etheridge RL, Herrera JR, Barry KL, Lynn N. Screening and brief intervention for substance misuse among older adults: the Florida BRITE project. Am J Public Health. 2010;100(1):108–14.
67. Center for Substance Abuse Treatment. Brief interventions and brief therapies for substance abuse; Treatment Improvement Protocol (TIP) Series 34. Rockville: Substance Abuse and Mental Health Services Administration; 1999.
68. Zanjani F, Davis T, Kruger T, Murray D. Mental health and aging initiative: intervention component effects. Rural and Remote Health. 2012;12:2154.

Index

A

Absorption, drug administration, 54
Acceptance and commitment therapy (ACT), 147–148
Acetaminophen
 characteristics, 124
 considerations for older adults, 125–126
 indications for use, 124–125
 mechanism of action, 124–125
 route of administration, 125
Activities of daily living (ADLS), 22
Acute herpes zoster, management strategies, 84
Acute pain
 management
  in emergency department, 38–39
  in medical inpatients, 44–46
  in nursing home, 46–48
  quality improvement in, 48–49
 prevalence and impact of, 35–36
Agency for Health Care Policy and Research (AHCPR) lists, 96
Age-related physiologic changes, 53
Aging, pharmacologic changes with, 73
American Geriatrics Society (AGS), 17
American Medical Directors Association (AMDA), 17
American Pain Society (APS), 94
American Society of Anesthesiologists (ASA), 42
Antiepileptic drugs, 127–130
Arthritis Foundation Self Help Program (ASHP), 6

B

Baby boomer population, 178
Behavioral interventions
 fear avoidance, 146
 operant behavioral therapy, 145–146
Benzodiazepine duration of action, 57
Biofeedback training, 143
Buprenorphine, 117

C

Cancer pain
 anti-cancer treatments, 80
 brain metastasis, 78
 etiologies, 76
 goals of care for patients, 77
 intractable pain, 80
 multimodal therapy, 80
 neuropathic pain, 77
 opioids for, 78
 post-chemotherapy pain, 80
 prevalence, 76
Caregiver self-assessment questionnaire, 21–22
Central pain processing disorders, clinical consequence, 97
Central post-stroke pain (CSP)
 causes, 103
 characteristics, 104
 goals of care, 104
 interventional therapies, 105
 management of, 104
 neurosurgical procedures, 106

Checklist of Nonverbal Pain Indicators (CNPI), 17
Chronic pain
  in aging populations, 132
  characteristics, 131
  prevalence of, 132
Codeine, 113
Cognitive-behavioral interventions
  acceptance and commitment therapy (ACT), 147–148
  cognitive-behavioral therapy (CBT), 146–147
  technological applications of, 148–149
Cognitive-behavioral therapy (CBT), 146–147
Complimentary therapies
  electrical nerve stimulation (ENS), 149
  massage therapy, 150
Compression fractures
  causes, 91
  diagnosis, 91
  goals of care, 91
  kyphoplasty/vertebroplasty, 92
  wedge fractures, 91
Consensus Panel of the Treatment Improvement Protocol (TIP), 186
Continuous intrathecal analgesia, 165–170
Contractures
  causes, 92
  complementary and alternative medicine techniques, 93
  extremity, 92
  goals of care, 93
  treatment, 93

D

Degenerative disorders, definition, 86–97
Degenerative joint disease (DJD). *See* Osteoarthritis (OA)
Delirium, perioperative pain and, 43–46
Dementia, treatment strategy for elderly with, 31
Diabetes mellitus, 76
Diphenylheptane derivates, 112
Disuse atrophy, 92
Drug abuse screening test (DAST), 183
Drug addiction
  4Cs, 181
  assessment, 181–184
  cannabis, 178
  clinical presentation, 180–181
  four A's, 183
  interview process, 183
  marijuana, 178
  opioids, 178
  prevalence by age, 178
  prevention, 187–188
  risk stratified management, 185–187
  tolerance, 181
  treatment, 185–187
Drug adverse effects, 59
Drug interactions, 60–64

E

Electrical nerve stimulation (ENS), 149–150
Epidural steroid injections, lumbar spinal stenosis, 154–155
Equianalgesic doses, 79
Excretion, 58
Exercise, 149

F

Facet joint
  injections and radiofrequency ablation, 155–159
  level of L4-L5, 158
Fear avoidance, 145–146
Fentanyl, 116
Fibromyalgia (FM)
  definition, 98
  goals of care, 98
  pharmacotherapy, 98
  pharmacotherapy for, 99
  prevalence, 98

G

Geriatric depression scale (GDS), 25, 139

H

Hepatic impairment patients, 68
Herpes Zoster. *See* Varicella zoster virus (VZV)
Hip fractures, 42
Hydrocodone, 114
Hydromorphone, 114
Hydrophylic drugs, 55

I

Instrumental activities of daily living (IADL), 22, 23

Interlaminar epidural steroid injection, fluoroscopic image of, 155
Intra-articular peripheral joint injections, 170–171
Intramuscular absorption, 55
Intrathecal analgesia
    characteristics of patients with cancer, 169
    contraindications to delivery system, 170
    pump system, 168
Intravenous absorption, 55

K
Kyphoplasty, 163

L
Levorphanol, 115
Lipophilic drugs, 55
Low back pain (LBP)
    definition, 94
    evaluation, 95
    goals of care, 97
    non-musculoskeletal cause, 96
    pyriformis syndrome, 96
    red flag, 95
    treatment options, 97
    yellow flag factors, 95
Lumbar spinal stenosis, 154–157

M
Massage therapy, 150
Medtronic Synchromed II intrathecal pump, 169
Mental healthiness and aging initiative (MHAI) intervention, 188
Meperidine, 115
Metabolism, 56–57
Methadone, 115
Mindfulness-based therapy, 144
Minimum Data Set (MDS), 46
Morphine, 113
Myofascial pain, 86

N
Neuromodulation, 165–166
Neuropathic pain, 134
Neuropathic Pain Special Interest Group (NeuPSIG), 76
Nociceptive and neuropathic pain, 133–134

Nonsteroidal anti-inflammatory drugs (NSAIDs), 122
    characteristics, 120
    common side effects of, 124
    considerations for older adults, 123–124
    indications for use, 121–123
    mechanism of action, 121
    pharmacokinetics, 121–123
    routes of administration, 123

O
Operant behavioral therapy, 145–146
Opioid risk tool (ORT), 183
Opioids
    age-specific considerations, 118–119
    characteristics, 110
    choice of, 111–112
    classification of, 79
    dosing considerations, 119–120
    indications for drug, 111
    long-acting, 79
    mechanism of action/classification, 110
    and metabolite half-lives, 56
    and nonsteroidal anti-inflammatory drugs (NSAIDs), 120
    routes of administration, 111
    short-acting, 79
    types of, 112–119
Oral absorption, 55
Oral opioid dosing chart, 79
Osteoarthritis (OA)
    cause of pain, 87
    characteristic X-ray findings, 88
    degree of disability, 87
    diagnosis, 87
    goals of care, 88
    nonpharmacologic therapies, 88
    opioids for, 89
    pathophysiology, 87
    pharmacologic agents, 88
    physical therapy, 88
    prevalence, 170
    risk factors, 87
    treatment, 89
Osteoporosis (OS), definition, 91
Oxycodone, 114

P
Pain
    6 A's, 31

Pain (cont.)
    assessment and management, 4–5
    cancer, 3
    cancer-related, 2
    characteristics, 1
    definition, 1
    diseases causing, 19
    epidemiology, 1–3
    in later life, 3–4
    management approaches in older adults, 5–8
    minority aging, 141
    nonpharmacologic therapies, 5
    opioids for chronic, 7
    pharmacologic therapies, 5
    in post-operative setting, 3
    prevalent causes in later life, 2
    treatment, pharmacotherapy, 141–142
Pain assessment
    caregiver assessment, 20–22
    cognitive assessment, 22–24
    documentation, 30
    in elderly, challenges of, 14
    emotional assessment, 24
    functional assessment, 22, 135
    hierarchy of, 17
    history, 15
    management implications, 29–30
    medication, 19
    nociceptive and neuropathic pain, 133–134
    in nonverbal patients/patients with advanced dementia, 30
    past medical history (PMH), 18–19
    perception and, 53–54
    physical examination, 24
    purpose of, 14
    red flags, 28
    tools, 37
        self-report instruments, 135–137
    vitamin D deficiency, 24
Pain Assessment in Advanced Dementia (PAINAD), 17
Pain behaviors
    in cognitively impaired elderly persons, 18
    noncommunicative patients and observation of, 137–138
Pain management
    approach to, 14
    Beer's list, 65
    of fracture/surgery related, 39–43
    in hospital, 39–42
Painful diabetic peripheral neuropathy (PDPN)
    goals of care for patients, 81
    incidence of, 80
    nonpharmacologic treatment options, 82
    pharmacologic treatments for, 82
    prevalence, 81
    signs and symptoms, 81
    treatment, 82
Patient Health Questionnaire (PHQ-9), 26
Perioperative pain and delirium, 43–46
Persistent postsurgical pain (PPSP)
    causes, 99
    goals of care, 100, 103
    hydromorphone, 101
    intractable forms of, 103
    morphine, 101
    post-op confusion, 99
    treatment, 100
Personality traits and pain, 138
Pharmacodynamic drug interactions, 60–64
Pharmacodynamics, 58–60
Pharmacokinetic drug interactions, 60–63
Pharmacokinetic interactions, analgesics, 61–62
Pharmacokinetics, 54–56
Phenanthrene derivatives, 112
Polymethyl methacrylate (PMMA), 161
Polymyalgia rheumatic (PMR)
    characteristics, 84
    diagnosis, 85
    etiology, 84
    and giant cell arteritis (GCA), 85
    goals of care, 86
    treatment, 86
Postherpetic neuralgia, treatment, 85. *See* Varicella zoster virus (VZV)
Postsurgical pain, opioid options for, 102
Pressure ulcers
    causes, 93
    goals of care for, 93
Protein-bound drugs, 56
Psychological functioning
    beliefs about pain, 140
    mood and emotional responses, 138–140
    personality traits, 138–139

R

Red flags, 28
Relaxation training, 144
Renal impairment patients, 67
Researched Abuse, Diversion and Addiction-Related Surveillance system (RADARS), 179

S

Sacroiliac joint, 160
Sacroiliac joint interventions, 159–161
Sciatica, 155–157
Screener and opioid assessment for patients with pain (SOAPP), 183
Screening Tool for Addiction Risk (STAR), 183
Self-regulatory interventions
  biofeedback training, 143
  mindfulness-based therapy, 144
  relaxation training, 144
Serotonin-norephinephrine reuptake inhibitors (SNRI), 126–127
  dosing and side effects, 128
Spinal cord stimulation (SCS)
  lead placement, 167
  probability of pain reduction, 167
Spinal stenosis
  cause, 90
  clinical presentation, 90
  diagnosis, 90
  goals of care, 90
  physical therapy, 90
  treatment options, 90
State-Trait Anxiety Inventory (STAI), 139
Sublingual absorption, 54–55
Substance abuse (SA)
  causes of, 179
  early-onset users, 179
  elderly population, 184
  late-onset users, 179
  patterns of use, 179
  risk factors for, 180
  treatment admissions, 178
Substance Abuse and Mental Health Services Administration (SAMHSA), 186
Substance use disorders (SUD), assessment of, 181
SynchroMed® Infusion System, 168

T

Tapentadol, 118
Tolerance, 181
Tramadol, 117
Transdermal adsorption, 54
Transforaminal epidural steroid injection, fluoroscopic image of, 156
Tricyclic antidepressants (TCA), 126–127
  dosing and side effects, 128

U

Urine drug testing (UDT), 182

V

Varicella zoster virus (VZV)
  acute zoster pain, 83
  analgesic agents, 84
  antiviral medication, 84
  characteristics, 83
  corticosteroid treatment, 84
  goals of care, 83
  incidence, 83
  management strategies, 84
  treatment, 83
Vertebral augmentation, 159–165
  contraindications to, 164
Vertebral compression fractures (VCFs), 91
Vertebroplasty
  and balloon kyphoplasty, 161–165
  needle placement for, 161
  polymethyl methacrylate under fluoroscopy during, 162

W

Wong-Baker FACES pain rating scale, 16

Z

Zarit Burden interview, 20

MIX
Papier aus verantwortungsvollen Quellen
Paper from responsible sources
FSC® C105338

If you have any concerns about our products,
you can contact us on
ProductSafety@springernature.com

In case Publisher is established outside the EU,
the EU authorized representative is:
**Springer Nature Customer Service Center GmbH
Europaplatz 3, 69115 Heidelberg, Germany**

Printed by Libri Plureos GmbH
in Hamburg, Germany